Temple Grandin

Temple Grandin

VOICE FOR THE VOICELESS

ANNETTE WOOD

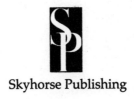

Skyhorse Publishing

Skyhorse Publishing books may be purchased in bulk at special discounts for sales promotion, corporate gifts, fund-raising, or educational purposes. Special editions can also be created to specifications. For details, contact the Special Sales Department, Skyhorse Publishing, 307 West 36th Street, 11th Floor, New York, NY 10018 or info@skyhorsepublishing.com.

Skyhorse® and Skyhorse Publishing® are registered trademarks of Skyhorse Publishing, Inc.®, a Delaware corporation.

Visit our website at www.skyhorsepublishing.com.
10 9 8 7 6 5 4 3 2 1

Library of Congress Cataloging-in-Publication Data is available on file.

Cover design by Rain Saukas

Print ISBN: 978-1-5107-0660-6
Ebook ISBN: 978-1-5107-0662-0

Printed in the United States of America

To Robert and Evelyn Nunemaker, my parents

CONTENTS

PART I

TEMPLE

CHAPTER 1

TEMPLE'S BEGINNINGS

Temple Grandin flies all over the world—to countries as diverse as Germany, China, and Uruguay. Her awkward stride, Western outfits, and unforgettable voice make her easily recognizable. She's renowned worldwide as a speaker, has written many books—two on the *New York Times* best-seller list—and has educated a new generation. This woman, who had to be taught how to talk, has given voice to two formerly voiceless groups: animals and people with autism. For those with autism who *can* talk, Temple has added greatly to our understanding of the condition. She's also contributed a great deal to our understanding of animals. Her insights into animal awareness are fascinating and groundbreaking.

Born with a disability severe enough that, had she been born into different circumstances, it would have required her to be institutionalized, Temple Grandin turned her disability into an asset. Her story is one of profound courage and determination.

Temple Grandin came from remarkable stock on both sides of her family.

Her paternal great-grandfather, John Livingston Grandin, made a fortune in oil, wheat, and the lumber business. His son, Temple's paternal grandfather, was also named John Livingston Grandin. He married Isabel McCurdy and moved to Boston where they had three children: Isabella in 1908, Richard McCurdy in 1914, and John Livingston in 1918. The middle child, Richard (Dick) Grandin, was Temple's father.

On her mother's side, Temple's grandfather, John Coleman Purves, married Mary Temple Bradley. Their child and Temple's mother, Anna Eustacia Purves, was born in September 1926. She was named after her maternal grandmother, yet was always called "Eustacia."

Temple's grandmother Mary always focused on being social while her husband John was a busy engineer and aviation expert. Though they loved each other, in many ways they were hopelessly mismatched.

During the 1930s, John and three other men invented an electrical coil that could sense direction through the earth's magnetic north. The four men named it the "flux valve." Later, the Army Air Corps called it "the automatic pilot" and flew their World War II planes by it. "After World War II, it took us all the way to the moon," Eustacia later said. Documents concerning the invention are in the Smithsonian.[1]

Both Grandfather Grandin and Grandfather Purves, though extremely intelligent, had social deficits. Little did they know how the genes of the four grandparents would collide in their granddaughter Temple.

In June 1944, Eustacia met Dick Grandin at the Boston Cotillion. It was Dick Grandin's thirtieth birthday and Eustacia was seventeen, only twenty-four hours out of a girls' boarding school. Isabella Grandin arranged for her brother Dick, an officer in the tank corps, to accompany Eustacia. Her father had refused to escort his daughter. Dick and Eustacia made an enchanting couple. The next morning their photo graced the society page.

Dick had graduated from Harvard, where he lived outside the dorms in a separate rented house with a manservant. One of his fellow clubmen was Johnny Roosevelt. Johnny invited them all to Sunday night supper at the White House where, Eustacia recalled, Mrs. Roosevelt scrambled eggs for them in a silver chafing dish brought in by the maid and lighted ceremoniously. After supper, Gershwin played them "Rhapsody in Blue."[2]

After Dick and Eustacia met came three days of telephone calls, flowers, and "girlfriend envy." Dick then departed for duty overseas, where he announced by mail that he planned to marry Eustacia.[3]

Dick fought in the Battle of the Bulge, a brutal, bloody battle. On December 16, 1944, in northern France the Germans, who by that time were losing the war, launched a desperate counterattack. Dick was a first lieutenant attached to a reconnaissance group.[4] War calls for courage, resourcefulness, and total obedience. Dick had an abundance of the first two, but lacked the third.

The battle lasted three weeks. Of the 610,000 Americans involved in the battle, 89,000 were casualties, including 19,000 killed. It was the bloodiest battle fought by the United States in World War II.[5] Dick had lived a privileged life until now. He was appalled at the death and destruction. He was convinced that the colonel above him was causing many of the casualties with his orders.

Dick chose to report the colonel to those in command, going over his commander's head to do so. The higher-ups warned him that if he made an official charge, the colonel's record would be kept "under wraps" and Dick would be moved to a different tank unit. In addition, Dick would have to forfeit his advancement from first lieutenant to major.[6]

Dick did it anyway and suffered the consequences. He did not become a major. Worse, he was separated from his old friends at a time when he could have used the support of established relationships. He told Eustacia, who concluded that he was very brave. Much later someone from Squadron A, of which Dick had been a part, told her, "We always knew Sticky Dick was crazy."[7]

Both families approved the engagement. Mary Purves, the socialite, was especially enthusiastic about her daughter making a good marriage. She found planning a wedding exhilarating. Dick and Eustacia were married in March 1946.

They had known each other less than two years. Dick had been away at war much of that time and had seen a lot of violence. He would have to make adjustments to civilian life. For as long as she had existed, Eustacia had been pampered. Since they had known each other such a short time, there must have been surprises—and difficulties—in living together. About eight months after their marriage, Eustacia became pregnant.

Eustacia was nineteen when Mary Temple, named after her maternal grandmother, was born on August 29, 1947. Her mother remembered her as a normal healthy newborn with big blue eyes, a mass of downy brown hair, and a dimple in her chin. One of the maids working for the Grandins at the time was named Mary, so to avoid confusion they called the baby Temple.

Eustacia, who only had one sister, had never held a baby or been around babies, so she knew little about being a mother. From the beginning, Temple showed no attachment to her mother, no playful responses. She didn't put things in her mouth. She objected to cuddling. She seemed neither happy nor unhappy. Eustacia compared Temple to babies of her friends and felt uncomfortable.

Eustacia had lived a charmed life until her first child was born. She had money, intelligence, good looks, talent, and a proper upbringing. "It creeps up on you slowly that something's wrong," Eustacia said later. Admitting, even to yourself, that something's amiss takes even longer.

In May 1949, Temple's sister was born. To her parents' relief, she developed normally, making Eustacia keenly aware of Temple's deficits. By this time, Temple was twenty-one months old and still lost in her own world. When she played in the sandbox, she dribbled the sand through her fingers, absorbed only in what she was doing.

By the time she was two and a half, Temple was still not talking. She didn't even laugh. She was decidedly odd. Her father thought she was deficient. Eustacia protested, but knew there was something not right. She made an appointment for Temple with Dr. Bronson Caruthers, head of the Judge Baker Guidance Clinic in Boston.

When Temple was three and still not talking, Dr. Caruthers recommended that she come to the children's hospital for a ten-day visit and have an electroencephalogram (EEG). Temple was strangely indifferent to the hospital surroundings and her mother leaving her. However, she protested the EEG. "Her face turned scarlet. Her hair was soaked from flinging her head about. Finally, the anesthesia took over, her screams turned to hiccupping sobs, and she fell asleep."[8]

The EEG was normal. Why an EEG? The doctor, ahead of his time, wanted to rule out epilepsy. Though it would be years before specialists would officially connect autism and epilepsy, that connection would be key in deciding autism was bioneurological.

A hearing test was also normal. The doctor shook his shaggy head and suggested a speech therapist.

Temple said later, "I could understand what was being said, but I was unable to respond. Screaming and flapping my hands was my only way to communicate."

Dr. Caruthers recommended Mrs. Reynolds for both individual speech therapy and a small nursery school class. Mrs. Reynolds grabbed Temple's chin and showed her the difference between a "b" sound and a "p" sound. Temple went to see her three times a week. Mrs. Reynolds was charming, and Temple loved her.

In the winter of 1951, Temple's new doctor diagnosed her with infant schizophrenia, which we now call autism. Almost nothing was known about autism at that time. It was thought to be a rare disorder, although it undoubtedly had been around for hundreds of years. Dr. Leo Kanner, director of Child Psychiatry at Johns Hopkins University, had identified autism in 1943— less than a decade before Temple was found to have it.

After Temple was diagnosed, Dick Grandin felt justified in his desire to institutionalize her. Eustacia was devastated. She wept uncontrollably. "It's easy to be overwhelmed," she would later tell others. "I vowed not to cry so hard again. I would listen only to those worth listening to."

In defense of Dick, doctors at the time often recommended institutions for children with behavior as extreme as Temple's, and people in that era tended to follow a doctor's orders. Though he resented spending money in this way, Dick wanted to put his daughter in an institution.

Eustacia was totally against it. Not surprisingly, this caused conflict between them. What is surprising is that this nineteen-year-old first-time mother stood up to a husband twelve years older than she, a man she considered smart and sophisticated. She fought for her child.

Temple was fortunate to have an early intervention, which would later become the biggest recommendation for a successful outcome with autism. She had twenty hours a week of speech therapy, nursery school, and a nanny who had worked with a boy whose behavior was similar to Temple's. The nanny played lots of board games with Temple and her sister, teaching them to take turns.

Eustacia also worked with them on taking turns. "Mother'd take one sled out on the hill and she'd make my sister and I take turns on that sled. Even at a young age, she was playing tiddlywinks with us," said Temple.[9]

Much later, Temple, nonverbal at the time but obviously aware, said, "I can remember a time when I was in speech therapy in nursery school. The teacher was using a blackboard pointer to point to the students to do something, and I was just screaming every time she aimed the pointer at me. I screamed because I was taught at home that you should never point an object at a person because it could poke out your eye. I could not tell the teacher that I was taught at home not to point things at people."

Eustacia was relieved and rejoiced mightily when Temple, who now was almost four, began talking. Not just single words, but whole sentences. Though her voice was flat with little inflection and no rhythm, she was talking.

Both Mrs. Reynolds and the social worker from the school system felt she was ready for a month at St. Hubert's, a camp for special children run by Mrs. Huckle, an Englishwoman.

Mrs. Huckle accepted Temple on the condition that by the end of the summer she has "learned two things, to say the Lord's Prayer and always do your veddy, veddy best."[10]

"Mrs. Huckle was not impressed by Temple's father," said Eustacia. "That impacted me." Eustacia also discovered the existence of a teacher network. One good teacher will likely recommend others.

At age five, Temple entered regular kindergarten in a small private school, Valley Country Day School. The brick and cinder block school stood at the heart of seventeen acres of fields and woods. It was less than a mile from the Grandin family home.

From an adult perspective Temple remembers, "The school had highly structured old-fashioned classes with strict rules, enforced consistently with consequences for infractions. The environment was quiet and controlled, without a high degree of sensory stimulation."[11] The school was typical of many schools in the 1950s.

Eustacia talked with Everett Ladd, the headmaster, and Mrs. Dietsch, the teacher for the first three grades. She explained Temple's story. Mr. Ladd requested that they stay in close communication and Mrs. Dietsch asked, "If Temple has a bad day, may we send her home?"

Eustacia readily agreed. Like most parents in that era, she expected good behavior from Temple, much to Temple's advantage. "Expectation and consistency between home and school is a must," Temple would say years afterward.

Eustacia proved extraordinary. "Mother was ahead of her time. She assumed she couldn't do anything about the cause of my behavior, so she concentrated on the behavior itself," said Temple.

Unlike many parents, Eustacia had access to a great deal of money, which she spent on psychiatrists, doctors, tests, private schools, speech therapists, and nannies. She also had determination to help her child and a spirit of adventure.

In her grade school years, though decidedly different with her flat monotone voice, inability to read social cues, and frequent tantrums, Temple was very much a part of school and community life. The community provided a shelter for her. The mothers had an informal agreed-upon code of behavior all of them expected from every child. And Temple was no exception.

Temple proved she could follow the rules. "When I was ten years old, I rode my bike everywhere and always obeyed the rules."[12]

When Temple had difficulties learning to read, Eustacia helped her. Eustacia chose *The Wizard of Oz* to engage her daughter in reading. Temple was enchanted with the pictures. Eustacia read some of it to her and then asked her daughter to read a paragraph. Before long, Temple was so caught up in the story, she read more than asked.

Eustacia spent thirty minutes a day, five days a week teaching Temple to read. After Eustacia worked with her, Temple did well on her elementary reading tests. "She got me engaged in reading in a way that was meaningful until reading became naturally reinforcing on its own," said Temple.[13]

Eustacia was good at emphasizing Temple's strengths. "When Mother had me sing at an adult concert when I was in sixth grade, I felt good about that."[14]

Especially good at art, Temple loved creating things. Her room was filled with creations of cardboard, string, and paint. "I started designing things as a child, when I was always experimenting with new kinds of kites and model airplanes," Temple recalled. "In elementary school, I made a helicopter out of a broken balsa-wood airplane. When I wound up the propeller, the helicopter flew straight up about a hundred feet. I also made bird-shaped paper kites, which I flew behind my bike. The kites were cut out from a single sheet of heavy drawing paper and flown with thread. I experimented with different ways of bending the wings to increase flying performance. Bending the tips of the wings up made the kite fly higher. Thirty years later, this same design started appearing on commercial aircraft."[15]

When her school had a pet show, Temple took herself. "I dressed up like a dog. I even had masters—the Reese twin boys. I performed like a dog—barking, sitting up, and laying down. I was a big hit and was rewarded with a blue ribbon."[16]

From an early age, Temple craved being touched, though she stiffened even when her mother hugged her. She daydreamed about a comfort device. "The advantage of a comfort device would be that I could control the amount of stimuli. I could satisfy my craving for comfort without flooding my senses with massive amounts of input my nervous system couldn't tolerate."[17]

Though she couldn't communicate about them at the time, Temple was distracted by sensitivities that most children don't have. For instance, she didn't like scratchy petticoats. She said they were like "sandpaper scraping at raw nerve endings." Like many autistic children, she was overly responsive to smells. "Several autistic people have told me that they remember people by smell and one reported that he liked safe smells like pots and pans, which he associated with home," Temple said.

Temple especially hated loud, unexpected noises, like balloons popping. Imagine birthday parties. "When the governess discovered that I didn't like loud noises, she punished me when I was bad by popping a paper bag in my ear," she remembered. "Torturing should never be used as a punishment."

Things other children barely noticed terrified Temple. "One night it rained really hard and the roof leaked, leaving a small water stain in my room. I feared the ceiling would collapse. The pictures conjured up in my visual mind were of all the upstairs furniture crashing down on me."

She had a common symptom of autism: fixations. In fourth grade, Temple had one that nearly drove her family crazy. "I talked constantly about election posters, buttons, and bumper stickers. I was fixated on the election of our state governor. All I talked about was his election to office."[18] Sometimes the other children told Temple that she was a pest.

She constantly asked questions and then repeated them. "I'd ask the same question and wait for the same answer— over and over again. If a particular topic intrigued me, I zeroed in on that subject and talked it to the ground."[19]

"We aren't good at conversation," said Naoki Higashida, a thirteen-year-old Japanese boy who wrote about his autism. "We'll never speak as effortlessly as you do. We can repeat words or phrases we're familiar with. It's great fun. It's like a game of catch with a ball. Repeating questions we already know the answers to can be a pleasure—it's playing with sound and rhythm."[20]

Temple has always had strong visualization skills, making her atypical. "I think in pictures. Words are like a second language to me. I translate both spoken and written words into full-color movies, complete with sound, which run like a VCR tape in my head. When somebody speaks to me, the words are instantly translated into pictures."

For many years, Temple was unaware that others do not usually think in pictures. She also didn't realize that she couldn't read social signals; she missed all the nonverbal communication that passed between "neurotypical" (people who do not have a developmental disorder such as autism) human beings automatically. "Something was going on between the other kids, something swift, subtle, constantly changing—an exchange of meanings, a negotiation, a swiftness of understanding so remarkable that sometimes I wondered if they were all telepathic."

In the fifties, no one talked about autism. "I myself didn't hear the word 'autistic' applied to me until I was about twelve or thirteen. I remember thinking, 'Oh, it's me that's different.'"

It's remarkable that Temple functioned as well as she did in grade school.

CHAPTER 2

MIDDLE SCHOOL AND HIGH SCHOOL

Autism, a complex neurological disorder, always appears before the age of three. The most common symptoms are: no speech or abnormal speech, lack of eye contact, frequent temper tantrums, oversensitivity to touch, appearance of deafness, a preference for being alone, rocking or spinning, aloofness, and lack of social contact with parents and siblings.

People with autism can be brilliant, have average intelligence, or intellectual disabilities.

Asperger's syndrome is related to social deficits/behavior domain. People with Asperger's have normal or advanced speech and language. Those with Asperger's often have exceptional intelligence, but lack a sense of social exchange and empathy.

When Temple went to junior high, she no longer fit in. "I couldn't figure out why I was having a problem with other kids. I had an odd lack of insight that I was different, probably because what I did was more meaningful to me than outward appearance," Temple recalls.

Temple graduated from Valley Country Day School, a private elementary school, which had only thirteen students and one teacher in her grade. Then she entered seventh grade at the Cherry Hill Girls School in Norwich, Connecticut, a school for upper middle-class girls. Like most junior high schools, it had thirty to forty students in a class and a different teacher for every class.

Neurotypical people frequently find the adjustment to junior high very stressful. This was magnified for Temple. A change in routine can cause an autistic person to have a tantrum. Now Temple faced multiple changes each hour. Not surprisingly, she melted down frequently. When Temple threw a history book at a fellow student and hit her in the eye, she was expelled.

In January 1960, twelve-year-old Temple arrived at Hampshire Country School in Rindge, New Hampshire, which had only thirty-two students when she enrolled. It was a boarding school for gifted, emotionally disturbed children. Other students besides Temple were probably autistic. Autism was not a word that was heard in the 1960s. Even professionals didn't use it. The second edition of the *Diagnostic and Statistical Manual of Mental Disorders* (DSM), published in 1968, did not mention autism.

Hampshire Country School was founded by Henry Patey, a psychologist, and his wife Adelaide, a teacher. They considered kids like Temple not bad or stupid, but possibly gifted or just misunderstood. Surrounded by 1,700 acres of woods and streams, Hampshire had not only classrooms, but a working dairy, sheep pens, and a stable with horses. Other extras included arts, crafts, camping, and canoe trips.

"Horseback riding was joyous for me," said Temple. "I can remember being on a horse sometimes and we'd gallop in the pasture and that was such a thrill. Or we'd be out on a trail riding, and do a really fast gallop down the road. I remember what it looked like, the trees whizzing by; I remember that really well to this day."[1]

Temple was so wrapped up in horses, she spent every spare moment working in the barns. "I was dedicated to keeping the barns clean, making sure the horses were groomed," she said.

At Hampshire, the principal took away the privilege of riding to discipline her when she smacked a fellow student. Temple was crushed when she couldn't ride. This encouraged her to behave.

Temple said, "When I was on horses, I got away from bullying—no texts, no phone calls. Kids couldn't do that today." (There were no texts or cell phones in Temple's day, but there were when she made this comment.)

Temple could tell when a horse started to get nervous by the swishing tail, becoming more rapid with mounting fear. She noticed the same details that the horses did, such as a bale slightly out of place. She could make small changes to calm the animal's fear before it turned to panic, demonstrating the ability to read animals that would make her famous.

As with most autistics, Temple craved sameness. "I even wore the same jacket and dressed in the same kind of clothes day in and day out."[2] For this reason, she adjusted slowly to boarding school—a definite switch from her home environment of three younger siblings and two parents. However, there were many things she enjoyed at school, including skiing, riding horses, and participating in horse shows. She worked hard to make costumes for the school play. She helped workmen shingle a new house and was proud of the results.

Temple had a blind roommate in high school. Her roommate didn't want a guide dog to lead her. She needed to be walked through a new environment only once, then she knew her way. Temple admired her roommate for her ability to cope with blindness.

Temple and her roommate got along, but getting along with others continued to be a problem. "When I was a teenager, I was aware that I did not fit in socially, but I was not aware that my method of visual thinking and my overly sensitive senses were the cause of my difficulties in relating to and interacting with other people."[3]

She didn't realize how other people saw her. Her inability to read social signals was a major handicap. Consider that slightly more than 90 percent of communication among people is nonverbal. For instance, she did not know that not returning a smile puzzled people. She did not look into the eyes of someone who was speaking. She did not know that tears rolling down a face usually meant sadness, although it could mean joy.

Curtly honest, Temple said what she thought without trying to soften her remarks. Although she didn't mean to, she often sounded abrupt and abrasive. She hesitated frequently and had a flat tone to her speech. She liked to repeat words and phrases. Much later, she concluded that speech therapy would have helped her much more than seeing a psychiatrist, which she had done in elementary school.

When Temple reached adolescence, raging hormonal changes swept over her. With them she developed panic attacks; fixations became her way to relieve the anxiety. Obsessions are great motivators. William Carlock, Temple's science teacher, channeled her fixations into constructive projects. As a NASA scientist, he taught her that science is doing, building, creating. He made science fun and exciting. As an adult, Temple would stress the importance of mentors for people with Asperger's.

"After seeing an illusion called Ames Trapezoid Window, I wanted to build one," said Temple. Mr. Carlock encouraged Temple to try it, giving her a glimpse in a textbook of how to do it. "He gave me a hint without telling me exactly how to do it. He helped me develop problem solving skills."[4]

Temple often found refuge in Mr. Carlock's science lab. He encouraged and mentored her. "Teaching a person with autism the social graces is like coaching an actor for a play," Temple said. "Mr. Carlock did more for me than teach me science. He spent hours giving me encouragement when I became dejected by all the teasing from classmates."[5]

Mr. Carlock identified Temple's strengths in mechanics and engineering. He ran the model rocket club and got her interested in all kinds of electronic experiments. But he wouldn't let her skip algebra and move on to geometry. He didn't understand that Temple's brain didn't work in the abstract. He didn't realize that she had limitations in that area. "Instead of ignoring deficits, you have to accommodate them," said Temple.[6] Along with not being able to work in the abstract, she can't balance on one foot, walk a chalk line, or do algebra.[7]

Hampshire Country School required chapel study, which usually bored Temple. She was apparently a typical teen in that regard. One Sunday, a loud knock interrupted her thoughts. The minister, who had knocked on wood to make a point, was preaching about doors: "I am the door, by me if any man enters, he shall be saved." The minister also talked about joy and love, which eluded Temple due to their abstraction.

Like most autistics, Temple took things literally. "For the next few days, I viewed each door as a possible opening to joy and love. The closet door, the bathroom door, the front door, the stable door—all were scrutinized and rejected as *the* door."[8]

Then she discovered another door. She found a ladder against a dorm that was in the process of being renovated, and she climbed up to the fourth floor. There she found a small platform and an entrance that opened out onto the roof.

"I stepped into a small observation room. There were three picture windows that overlooked the mountains." Temple decided she'd found her door to heaven. "In the days and months that followed, I visited the observation room or Crow's Nest, as the carpenters called it, often."[9]

In 1962, when Temple was a vulnerable adolescent, her parents divorced. Their relationship had deteriorated for years. Her sister Jean had long ago asked, "Do you think Mom and Dad will get a divorce?" Now it became a reality.

A marriage is complex and mysterious, and both sides play a part in its success or failure. Still, Dick Grandin would have been hard to live with. "Dad would blow up in restaurants if the food took too long to arrive. He also had a tendency to fixate on a single subject," said Temple about the infamous Grandin temper. "One time he got obsessed with shutting down the riding stable next door to his house. He spent days and days writing letters to the city officials and measuring the amount of manure that was thrown in the dumpster."[10]

Temple thinks her father had Asperger's. People with severe autism frequently have a family member or members with Asperger's, a mild form of autism, or dyslexia, also thought to be a form of autism.

Fortunately for Temple, her mother married Ben Cutler in 1965. Thus she inherited a number of relatives, including Ann Beecham, Ben's sister. Aunt Ann lived on a guest ranch in Arizona and invited Temple to spend the summer. Though Temple hesitated to go, the summer on a ranch in Arizona changed her life.

Her mother pushed her to go. She always wanted Temple to try new things. "I didn't want to go, but instead of letting me stay home, Mother told me if I didn't like it, I could go home in two weeks," Temple remembers.

Ann was patient with Temple in ways that few people had been. She listened as Temple repeated stories over and over. Ann suggested constructive ways to channel her energy and fixations. She encouraged Temple to do physical labor, which Temple had always been good at and enjoyed. For instance, she rebuilt the roof of the pump house and repaired a railing on the fence. She invented a device she called the Magic Gate: "All you had to do was pull a rope, which you could easily do from the driver's side window, and the gate would swing open. Weights attached to a pulley system would swing the gate shut after your car pulled through."[11]

Temple learned to drive on the dirt roads of Aunt Ann's ranch. She drove three miles to the mailbox every day all summer. The ranch pickup had a manual clutch, which didn't work quite right. Temple mastered both steering and the tricky clutch while Aunt Ann sat beside her. Her aunt made sure she gained command of steering, braking, and changing gears before she let Temple drive on a paved road with traffic.[12]

In Arizona, Temple discovered a world where she felt comfortable. She had horses to ride and found she related well to cows. At a neighboring ranch, Temple saw a herd of cattle being put through the squeeze chute, an apparatus used to hold still a cow for medical shots by squeezing her so tight she can't move. The squeeze chute looks like a big V made of metal bars hinged at the bottom. When a cow walks into the chute, an air compressor closes up the V, which squeezes the cow's body in place.

Temple had dreamed for years about a device she could control that would "hug" her. She coveted touch, but, like most autistics, shrank from it because "my nervous system does not have time to process the sensation." She would not even let her mother hug her.

She had built her life around avoiding anxiety attacks. When she noticed how a cow relaxed after being put into the squeeze chute, she decided she wanted to get into it. Finally she told her aunt, who agreed to let Temple try it.

"Ann pulled the rope, which pulled the sides of the squeeze chute together. Soon I felt the firm pressure on my sides. Ordinarily, I would have withdrawn from such pressure, but in the cattle chute, withdrawal wasn't possible. The effect was both stimulating and relaxing, but most important for an autistic person, I was in control. I was able to direct Ann to the comfortable degree of pressure. The squeeze chute provided relief from my nerve attacks."[13]

That summer Temple made her first connection between cows and herself. She also became addicted to the effects of the squeeze machine. When she returned to school, she built a crude replica of it. Unlike the rest of the school, Mr. Carlock did not scoff. "If you want to know why this relaxes you, you'll have to learn science," he said.

He took her to the library and showed her how to use the books that scientists used. Temple found the language of science and technology easy to understand. For Temple, technical language was far simpler than negotiating the world of irony, metaphors, allusions, and jokes. She studied hard so she could get into college and be a scientist. She had found a reason to study.

She used her fixation on the cattle chute with good results. She explained fixations this way. "Stubbornness is related to perseverance and perseverance is a good trait. The traits in an autistic are the same as the traits in a normal person, but in an autistic some of the traits have gone haywire."[14]

When she graduated from high school on June 12, 1966, she was chosen to give one of several speeches. Temple said, "In looking back on the door now, I realize that it represented my maturing and getting ready to graduate from high school. The unknown that lay beyond the door represented what was beyond high school for me. I had the typical teenager's question, 'Is there life after high school?'"

CHAPTER 3

FRANKLIN PIERCE COLLEGE

After her senior year in high school at Hampshire Country School, Temple again spent the summer in Arizona on her aunt's ranch. This time, she was with old friends, so she was much more relaxed.

The next fall, she entered Franklin Pierce College, a small college in New Hampshire in the same town as her high school. Franklin Pierce was surrounded by mountains, lakes, woods, and meadows. About four hundred students entered her freshman class. She was grateful for its relatively small size.

"Had I entered a large university, I would have been lost in the maze of many buildings and thousands of students," Temple said.

Best of all, she could still see Mr. Carlock, her mentor at Hampshire Country School. He knew how her mother and the school psychologist objected to her squeeze machine. "Well, let's build a better one and do some scientific experiments with college students," Mr. Carlock said. "Let's find out if the squeeze machine really does relax. Find out if the effect is indeed real."

"I spent hours at the library looking up everything I could find on the effect sensory input into one system had on sensory perception in another," Temple said. She found a world of information she didn't know existed. Then she built PACES, or Pressure Apparatus Controlled Environment Sensory. "This model with its foam-padded panels was a Cadillac compared to my first Spartan wooden chute," said Temple.

Next, Temple designed a psychology experiment in which she tested the squeeze machine on other college students. From the experiment, she found that twenty-five out of forty neurotypical college students who tried it found the squeeze machine to be pleasurable and relaxing. She later published a scientific paper about the results.

As Temple used it regularly, she noticed distinct changes in herself. "I speculated that the regular use of the squeeze machine may help change some of the abnormal biochemistry, caused by the lack of comforting tactile stimulation in my early childhood."

Gradually, she was able to accept a pat on the shoulder or a handshake. All her life, she had stiffened at such contact, even if it was brief. Now, she found herself able to respond a little.

In this era of Freudian thought, the staff, some of her friends, and even her mother suggested all kinds of sexual implications, which only made her feel guilty. Fortunately, she had Mr. Carlock to encourage her. She was on the way to discovering a soothing resource of help for autistics, who react to touch with "tactile defensiveness," or hypersensitivity. (Today, many classrooms for autistic children use the "hug machine.")

From her experience with the squeeze machine, she found she was able to feel for others. Slowly, she started to have feelings of empathy, usually lacking in autistics. "From the time I started using my squeeze machine, I understood that the feeling it gave me was one I needed to cultivate toward other people," Temple said.[1]

She credits the machine with helping her to develop empathy. When she uses it, her thoughts often turn to her mother, her favorite teachers, and others who've touched her life in a positive way. "I feel my love for them and their love for me."

While at Franklin Pierce College, Temple took a course on genetics from Professor Burns. He taught the model Gregor Mendel had developed in the nineteenth century. In this model each parent contributes half the genes to an offspring. Species gradually change through a long series of random genetic mutations. Temple knew that couldn't be the whole explanation for passing down traits. She gave the example of a Border collie and a springer Spaniel that bred. All the puppies looked like a mixture of the two breeds, but not exactly half and half.[2]

In my family, there are five children. None of us look or act alike. A teacher who had four of us marveled at how different we were. One time at a basketball game, somebody asked my mother if we all had the same father. Someone else leaned over and said, "Do any of your children have the same father?" We all have the same father, but apparently our parents had a wide variety of genes. The shortest child is five feet two inches, the tallest is six feet three and a half inches, and our coloring differs.

In the sixties while Temple attended college, things were happening in the autism community that would eventually affect everyone living with a person with autism. In 1967 Bruno Bettelheim's book, *The Empty Fortress: Infantile Autism and the Birth of the Self,* appeared in print. By 1969, Bettelheim's book had sold more than fifteen thousand hardcover copies—an impressive number for a book stating that autism was the parent's fault.

Bettelheim, who was regarded as one of the world's most important and influential psychotherapists, found an audience for his views. Unfortunately, his message was: "Throughout this book, I state my belief that the precipitating factor in infantile autism is the parent's wish that his child should not exist."[3] This view outraged parents of autistic children, but it prevailed for years.

Only later was it discovered that Bettelheim had falsified his credentials when he moved to the United States in 1939. (Richard Pollak, author of *The Creation of Doctor B: A Biography of Bruno Bettelheim*, publicized that Bettelheim had lied about his credentials, but not until 1997.)

My sister Jan was diagnosed with autism in 1958, a time when the general public had not heard about it. My parents didn't say much about it, but I remember my shock when I read the words "childhood schizophrenia," which was often used as an alternate to "infantile autism." I was nine when I read this in a report from Dr. Helmer Myklebust, who had evaluated Jan in Chicago. I can only imagine my parents' horrified reaction. It must have been similar to that of other parents whose child was diagnosed with autism at the time.

In 1967, Bernard Rimland, PhD, a professional research psychologist, founded the Autism Research Institute in San Diego, California. His son Mark, who was born in 1956, had screamed for hours every day as a baby and a toddler. He ignored his parents, but "rocked constantly in his crib, often banging his forehead on the headboard." Change infuriated the boy, and he threw frightening tantrums when his mother, Gloria, came near him in a new dress. She solved the problem by buying several dresses of the same pattern from Sears for herself, her mother, and her mother-in-law—the only people who were willing to cope with Mark's behavior.[4]

At the time, the idea that bad parenting caused autism still reigned. Not only were parents dealing with a child whose difficulties they didn't understand, they were being blamed for their behavior. Like other parents of autistic children, Dr. Rimland decided this made no sense, and he was in a position to disprove this theory. He started reading everything he could find on autism. And he started writing.

In 1964, Prentice Hall published Bernard Rimland's *Infantile Autism: The Syndrome and Its Implications for a Neural Theory of Behavior.* Dr. Rimland concluded that "no evidence existed to support that autism was caused by bad parenting."[5] He found significant research suggesting that autism was an organic disorder. As a professional research psychologist, Rimland was the first authoritative voice to dispute the "refrigerator mother" theory, which held that autism was the result of lack of maternal affection or warmth. (Rimland was familiar with Bettelheim's theories, though Bettelheim hadn't yet published his book.)

Now parents of autistic children had someone with clout to support what many already knew. Parents from all over the United States began to write to Dr. Rimland. Some of the families met in Teaneck, New Jersey, to discuss their concerns. From this group came the Autism Society of America.

The organization held its first annual meeting in 1969 on the July weekend when most of the nation was watching the moon landing. Neil Armstrong announced one giant leap for mankind at the same time that four hundred registrants were listening to presentations by leading authorities in the field of autism.[6]

Leo Kanner, who had discovered autism, was among them. He reminded the audience that since the 1940s he had suspected that autism had an organic base. He even commented "with feeling" that *I herewith especially acquit you as parents.*[7]

Temple's mother, though not in the audience, was definitely not a refrigerator mother. Temple's mother always told her daughter: "Be proud you're different. You'll achieve more."

And achieve Temple did. In the spring of 1970, she graduated from Franklin Pierce College. She credited the squeeze machine with her improvement in socializing. She worked on the school's talent show, constructing and painting almost half the sets. "It was easier to make contact with other people while doing an activity we all were interested in," said Temple.[8]

Temple wrote about her squeeze machine in a paper for her final essay in a marriage and family class. She wrote: "God, whatever that is, and chance formed the gene structure that made me, and something happened in the process which disconnected the 'wire' in the brain that attracts a child to its mother and other humans offering affection."[9]

She speculated that maybe God wanted it that way so she would invent something that helped other people with the same sensitivity to touch that she had.

Temple graduated with a B.A. in psychology, second in a class of four hundred. No one yet knew what an extraordinary gift she would be to the world.

CHAPTER 4

TEMPLE IN THE SEVENTIES

After Temple graduated from Franklin Pierce College, she returned to Arizona to work on her master's degree. All her life, she'd had a deep connection to animals and she hoped to work with them, but she entered Arizona State University for graduate work in psychology.

She wanted to do her master's thesis on the behavior of cattle in feedlots on different types of cattle chutes. Her adviser at Arizona State University didn't think that was an appropriate academic subject. This was the early 1970s and research on animal behavior was nearly nonexistent. Thanks to Temple, the animal-behavior field would soon be transformed—but no one knew that at the time.

She didn't discourage easily, but she had to find someone to advise her on her thesis. Temple found Dr. Foster Burton, chairman of the construction department, and Mike Nielson from industrial design. Both were interested and agreed to guide her.[1]

Temple was only in graduate school part-time. She also worked part-time as a cattle chute operator. The first time she went to a feedlot and operated a cattle chute on a hundred and thirty head of cattle with three other workmen was the hardest. The animals were given full treatment: branding, shots, and castration. She felt relieved when she didn't come unglued.[2] In fact, though she was a woman from a wealthy family in Boston, she felt like she belonged. "You're some worker," one of the men complimented her.

At the end of her second year in graduate school, Temple switched her major from psychology to animal science. By that time, she had spent much effort and energy visiting cattle feedlots and slaughterhouses in Arizona to learn how to design cattle-handling facilities.

Temple tuned in to cows and their feelings of fear and anxiety. She suspected her nervous system resembled a cow's, and she identified with them. By touching and reassuring them, she showed respect for the animals' feelings. She discovered she always knew when an animal was in trouble.

She demonstrated her strong feelings for cattle as she fed cows out of her hand and touched them affectionately. She often laid her head on a cow. "Pressure is calming to the nervous system of a cow or an autistic person," said Temple.

"Animal behavior was the right field for me, because what I was missing in social understanding I could make up for in understanding animals," she said. "Autism is a kind of way-station on the road from animals to humans."

She exhibited her comprehension of animals time and time again. "I credit my visualization abilities with helping me [to] understand the animals I work with. Early in my career, I used a camera to help give me perspective as they walked through a chute for their veterinary treatment."

Temple knelt and took pictures through the chute from the cow's eye level. No one had ever done that before. She discovered what the cows were afraid of: a discarded soda bottle, a shadow, a moving vehicle. This was an important find. Time and time again throughout her career, she would be called in to find out why cows refused to move.

According to Temple, "Details are extremely important. A huge amount of my consulting business is getting paid to see all the stuff normal people can't see.

"Animals and autistic people don't have to be paying attention to something in order to see it. Things like jiggly chains pop out at us and grab our attention whether we want them to or not."[3]

Few people had heard of autism in the 1970s. They only knew Temple radiated weirdness. She was "always hunched over, wrung her hands and had an excessively loud, unmodulated voice." She dressed inappropriately and her underarms stank, sometimes permeating the air around her. From her grade school days, people frequently called her "Tape Recorder" because she talked incessantly, repeating stories and phrases over and over.

Temple saw that her isolated social life was symbolically epitomized in an image of glass. "She was a graduate student in her twenties, washing the bay window of a cafeteria, which consisted of a series of glass sliding doors. Slipping between the two doors to clean them, Temple suddenly found herself trapped inside. 'It was almost impossible to communicate through the glass,' she writes. 'Being autistic is like being trapped like this.'"[4]

I did not meet Temple until the 1990s at a conference for parents and teachers dealing with autistic preschoolers. This was after she had a reputation as an expert in both the autism and animal behavior fields. Her ideas were good, but I was startled by her strangeness. I can only imagine the reaction of people in the 1970s who knew nothing about her.

Several mentors accepted Temple for who she was and guided her through the world of stockyards and meat-packing plants. "Tom Rohrer, the manager of the Swift meat-packing plants, and Ted Gilbert, the manager of the Red River Feedlot (John Wayne's Feedlot), allowed me to visit their operations every week. They recognized my talents and tolerated my eccentricities," she recalled.[5]

Emil Winnisky, the construction manager at Corral Industries, a large feedlot in Arizona, recognized Temple's talents and helped her dress more appropriately. He had one of his secretaries go shopping with her. He also plunked down a jar of Arid deodorant on Temple's desk and said to her, "Your armpits stink." Though Temple resented it at first, she later realized Winnisky had done her a favor.

While she was at the construction company, she learned drafting from Davy, a shy loner who drew beautifully. Davy gave her suggestions on the tools to use for drafting. Temple was a talented artist. With her extraordinary visual skills, she was able to see cows moving through the system in her head. She could rotate the image and make it move in her mind like a movie.

Temple always visualizes an object before she draws it. "When I'm drawing a blueprint, remodeling a plant or designing a project, my thinking starts with an image of the object. Even the movies in my head start with an object.

"I knew that drawing was not only what I could do, it was what I did best. I took what nature gave me and nurtured the heck out of it."[6]

At a rodeo, Temple walked up to the publisher of *Arizona Farmer Ranchman* and asked him if he'd be interested in an article on designs of various squeeze chutes. She knew that the story would enhance her reputation as an expert in this field. She was delighted when he said, "Yes."

Several weeks later she received a call from the magazine. They not only wanted to publish the article, they also wanted to take her picture in the stockyards. "It was plain old nerve that got me my first job," said Temple. "That was in 1972. From then on I wrote regularly for the magazine while finishing my master's degree."

Writing for *Arizona Farmer Ranchman* was a fantastic experience for Temple. "I had repeated opportunities to visit many different places to do stories and interacted with a lot of different people."[7]

By the time Temple earned her master's degree, people had started to listen to her. Her articles in *Arizona Farmer Ranchman* were widely read and admired. Temple also contributed a chapter to a book on feedlot design.

Many of the workers and managers taunted her as she broke into this formerly all-male world. Temple was an anomaly as a woman in the world of cowboys, construction workers, and slaughterhouse employees. The men decorated Temple's car with bull testicles. They showed her the blood pit on several occasions. Finally, Temple splattered blood all over the plant manager.

"I didn't know whether autism or being a woman was the bigger handicap," said Temple.

"You can't believe how hard it was for Temple," said Jim Uhl, president of Agate Construction Company in Scottsdale, Arizona. "I remember one guy said, 'I won't have any woman teach me how to do cattle facilities!'"

Temple finished her master's at Arizona State University in 1975, one of the first farm animal research projects in the world. Her work on cattle behavior and handling is considered pioneering in her field.

After Temple finished school, she visited twenty feed yards in Arizona and then more in Texas. She observed and worked cattle in about thirty feed yards. "One had a really nice curved lead-up chute and another a nice loading ramp, but terrible sorting pens. When I sat down to design, I threw out all the bad parts and kept all the good parts."

She began her freelance career by designing cattle chutes for Corral Industries, and gradually took on more jobs. "In the 1970s when I was first getting started with my cattle equipment design business, I always carried with me a portfolio of designs and drawings," she noted.[8] She made her first contacts by telephone because it was easier for her than meeting in person. She didn't have to deal with as many complex social signals. She got an opportunity from an outbreak of scabies in Arizona. Scabies, a skin disorder, is caused by mites who lay eggs beneath the animal's skin, creating a terrible itch. Scabies is extremely contagious. Cattle with lots of mites scratch so hard they lose their hair, get infections, and even lose their lives.

In the 1970s, there was only one way to treat scabies. Each animal had to be plunged up to their ears in a pool of pesticide in a dip vat. The cattle didn't want to go into a vat that was seven feet deep, which caused a big problem for the owners. One of the managers at Red River Feedyard asked Temple to design a dip vat that cattle wouldn't fear. Temple understood why they were frightened. "Those cattle must have felt [like] they were forced to jump down an airplane escape slide into the ocean," she wrote.[9]

By then Temple had studied, measured, and photographed cattle facilities for six years. Typical of Temple, she spent hours working on a design, carefully including elements she knew the cattle would like and discarding those she knew they wouldn't.

Temple created a concrete ramp instead of a metal one. She added deep grooves for sure footing. The cattle would enter the water in single file, but they still wouldn't go underwater. And yet the treatment wouldn't work if the pesticide didn't reach their ears.

Temple had to get creative to solve the problem. She angled the ramp steeply in order to create a drop-off. After the cattle plopped quietly into the water, which was over their heads, they bobbed quickly to the surface. "Cattle are good swimmers and effortlessly swam to the other side."[10]

The new dip vat was a great innovation; it was highlighted in regional and national farm and ranch magazines. Word spread. Temple's designs were revolutionary.

In 1975, Jim Uhl sought out Temple after learning about her designs. He hung out around the stockyards in Scottsdale and wanted to build cattle-handling facilities, but he, like everyone else, had no experience in designing them. He heard there was a young woman who had successfully planned some, and coaxed Temple into meeting him at a café. She was suspicious at first. Many men at the stockyards had treated her badly. Only gradually did she relax.

"There were no other designers then for livestock facilities," said Uhl.[11] Temple understood cattle like no one else, even if she was from the East. Even if she was a woman.

Temple learned to carefully choose new projects. "Developers must choose carefully companies with management that believes in what they are doing, and they need to inspect every detail. Early adapters must be supervised at every step of installation and startup to make sure that the new method works correctly," Temple wrote.[12]

Temple was fortunate to have met Jim Uhl, who treated her with respect and believed in her designs. Likewise, Jim's company, Agate Construction, flourished partly because of Temple. Her photo is on Agate Construction's corporate wall.

One of Temple's early clients was not completely satisfied with her work. Temple thought about giving up her freelance business as a result. "My black and white thinking led me to believe that clients would always be 100 percent satisfied. Fortunately, Jim Uhl wouldn't let me give up. He pushed me and kept asking for the next drawing. Now I know that 100 percent client satisfaction is impossible," she said.[13] Jim and his crews have built twenty of Temple's projects in eleven different states. Temple traveled and worked right alongside them. "I thought I was a hard worker," said Jim. "But Temple can outdo me. She works on whatever needs to be done, even dragging steel with the guys." And she works seven days a week, sometimes three months at a time.

In 1979 Temple, Jim, and his construction crew traveled to Boston to build a demonstration cattle-handling facility for the Massachusetts Society for Prevention of Cruelty to Animals. They created a farm complete with pigs, sheep, goats, and cows for schoolchildren to visit. City children have few opportunities to be exposed to animals, and this provided one.

Temple and Jim became lifelong friends, but she did not get along with all the men she worked with. It took work, but Temple learned to be tactful and diplomatic. She has learned never to go over the head of the person who hired her unless she has their permission.

"I quickly learned that I wouldn't keep a job for long if I refused to do work, or argued with my boss or co-workers over assignments," she wrote.[14]

"I caused trouble for Tom Rohrer after I wrote a letter to the president of Swift about a bad equipment installation, which caused cattle to suffer. The president was embarrassed. He felt threatened and told Tom to get rid of me," she recalled.[15]

Fortunately, Tom did not fire her. He recognized her good intentions. He knew she was technically right, but socially wrong. This is one of the reasons people with autism need mentors.

Temple adds: "I have learned to avoid situations where I could be exploited or my employers might feel threatened. I learned diplomacy by reading about international negotiations and using them as models." She recommends reading the *Wall Street Journal*. The paper's articles were extremely helpful in increasing her understanding of workplace dynamics, social/office etiquette, and even more nebulous topics like office politics.[16]

Like her great-grandfather, John Grandin, Temple saw opportunities and she grabbed them. Like him, she has the qualities of persistence and courage. Her success is an inspiration to all.

CHAPTER 5

TEMPLE IN THE EIGHTIES

Temple founded her own company, Grandin Livestock Handling Systems, in 1980. Her business grew out of her life-long fascination with cattle and her talent for drawing. She put the two together in forming her business. "I saw a need in the livestock industry that hadn't been met, the need for a more humane system of slaughtering cattle and producing meat for American consumers," said Temple.[1]

She designed the single file race (chute), the curved race (chute), stockyard pens, ramps for livestock, and cattle dip vats. She used her empathy with cows to design equipment for them. She designed a conduit for cows the way a hose is a conduit for water. She had observed that cows like to stay with the herd and that cattle follow a curved path more easily.

"There are two reasons for this: First, the cattle can't see what is at the other end and become frightened and, secondly, the curved equipment takes advantage of the animal's behavior," she observed.[2]

Her sense of animals' moods and feelings is strong. "When I'm with cattle, it's not at all cognitive," she noted. "I know what the cow's feeling."

Temple relaxes when she's with cows. She feels like she's surrounded by friends. She sits in the grass with them and feeds them bits of hay. She lies down and allows them to nuzzle her. She knows they're curious.

Temple imagines what it is like to experiencing things through the cow's sensory system. She places herself inside the cow's body and recreates what it feels.

Cattle have a wide, panoramic visual field, because they are a prey species, watchful and wary for signs of danger. Members of a prey species such as cattle or sheep have to flee when they spot a predator. Even though cattle and sheep today are usually in pastures or feedlots where they seldom have predators, they've retained this skill. Temple takes this into consideration when designing equipment for cattle.

Like Temple, cattle and sheep have acute hearing. "Farm animals have sensitive hearing and are sensitive to high-pitched sounds. They can hear high-frequency sounds that people cannot hear. The human ear is most sensitive to sounds in the 1000–3000 hz range and cattle and horses are most sensitive to frequencies at 8000 hz and above," she wrote.[3]

Temple says that cattle startle easily and are overly anxious. Both cows and persons with autism experience a great deal of fear. Temple has spent much of her life avoiding panic attacks. Beginning in adolescence, waves of sweaty-palmed, gut-wrenching, stomach-churning fear engulfed Temple constantly, restricting her diet to Jell-O and yogurt for days, because the panic attacks affected her intestines.

Along with soothing herself with her squeeze machine, she started taking medication—50 mg of Tofranil, generic name imipramine—in the 1980s to reduce her anxiety. She learned about it from an article in *Psychology Today*[4] and read scientific journal articles before she asked her doctor to put her on the medication.[5] Within a week, 90 percent of her anxiety and panic was gone.[6]

With the medication, she says, "I am more relaxed and get along better with people. Stress-related problems like colitis are gone."[7] She does not perseverate nearly as much: "Reducing anxiety helped to reduce perseveration."[8]

This does not mean that Tofranil is appropriate for everyone who has autism. Autistics are all individuals, varied in skills, interests, likes, and dislikes, and have differing nervous systems. Medication that works for one does not necessarily work for another.

Because she wanted contact with others like herself, Temple attended her first Autism Society of America (ASA) conference (which was then called the National Society for Autistic Children in the mid-1980s). She met Dr. Ruth Sullivan, parent of Joseph, an autistic child. Dr. Sullivan was the first president of NASC.*

Dr. Sullivan asked Temple if she'd be willing to speak at the next ASA annual conference, then the only national conference about persons with autism. She agreed.

At the next conference, Temple told the audience about her sound sensitivities. "It's like being tied to a railroad track and the train's coming," she said. On the topic of underwear, she described her profound skin sensitivity: "I don't have the

---

* Ruth Sullivan was one of the chief lobbyists for Public Law 94–142, the Education for All Handicapped Children Act, which was later revised and renamed as the Individuals with Disabilities Act (IDEA). This bill guarantees public education up to the age of twenty-one for all children in the United States. Before passage of this law, individual school districts in most states were allowed to choose whether they were willing to educate a child with disabilities.

words to tell you how painful it is."[9] She talked about how hard it was to communicate what she felt, and about her difficulty in understanding others.

At that time, answers to the puzzle of autism were largely undiscovered. Families ventured into the world of autism with little explanation, scant information, and poor understanding. Without answers, family life became more and more topsy-turvy. Disappointment, despair, and frustration seeped in as parents struggled with a child's autism. As neurotypical persons, the audience grabbed this opportunity for answers.

"Temple spoke from her own experience, and her insight was impressive. There were tears in more than one set of eyes that day," Dr. Sullivan remembered.[10]

After that, Temple began speaking regularly at autism conferences. At first, she was not a good speaker. "She didn't seem to be addressing the audience, had no eye contact, might actually be facing in another direction, and could not take questions after the lecture," noted famed neurologist Dr. Oliver Sacks.[11]

However, she persevered and continued speaking about autism. She was familiar with the scientific facts about autism and had personal experience. Lorna King, founder and CEO of the Children's Center for Neurodevelopmental Studies, spoke at conferences with Temple. She noted big improvements in Temple's presentations as she continued speaking to groups. King wrote to Temple after one conference, praising her progress: "At this conference, you handled questions easily, rubbed shoulders with the crowd during breaks, shook hands without hesitation, and generally seemed calm and self-assured."[12]

Buoyed and encouraged by King's praise, Temple continued to speak at both autism and animal behavior conferences and her skills increased even more.

An editor at Arena Press heard about Temple speaking to groups about autism and asked if she would write a book about her experiences. Since Temple had no writing experience at the time, Arena Press enlisted Margaret M. Scariano as her co-author. Their collaboration, entitled *Emergence: Labeled Autistic*, was published in 1986.

Dr. Bernard Rimland, director of the Autism Research Institute, wrote the foreword. He had written his own groundbreaking book, *Infantile Autism*, in 1964.

Dr. Rimland and his wife took Temple to lunch. He remembers, "Her loud, unmodulated voice, characteristic of autistic persons, brought puzzled stares from the other diners. I risked offending her by asking her several times to lower her voice. She wasn't offended. She was open, candid, and quite unembarrassed. Here was an individual who recognized that she had oddities and peculiarities of speech and manner as a result of her autism.

"Not only was Temple not offended, she knew that improvement was appropriate and needed. It's a pleasure to deal with a person so forthright and uninterested in guile."[13]

William Carlock, Temple's beloved science teacher from high school, composed the preface to her book. Carlock wrote: "Temple has demonstrated, without question, that there is hope for the autistic child—that deep, constant caring, understanding, acceptance, appropriately high expectations, and support and encouragement help him (or her) reach his potential."[14]

Temple's book was a sensation, since people with autism don't typically develop enough language to write a book. It was the first of many books she wrote or edited.

But Temple did not have a huge breakthrough in her ability to cope with autism. She took a series of incremental steps, including during her journey to her PhD.

Stan Curtis in the animal science department at the University of Illinois kept a spot open for Temple, who was weak in math ability, to study for her PhD in Animal Science.[15] In the early 1980s, she enrolled in the University of Illinois to study and work with Dr. Bill Greenough, who became her dissertation co-adviser.

Temple was interested in the differing effects between barren environments and stimulating environments and the welfare of pigs. She studied twelve pigs in a barren environment, with hard plastic floors. Twelve other pigs were in an enriched environment with lots of straw, plastic balls, old telephone books, and metal pipe. Every day Temple changed something. She discovered, "New straw is exciting, old straw is boring."[16] Pigs are obsessed with straw.

Pigs are also driven to explore their world. One pen of Temple's research pigs at the University of Illinois learned to unscrew the bolts that held the pen divider to the wall.[17] Temple screwed the bolts in and the pigs unscrewed them.

Greenough's neuroscience class opened up the world of brain research to Temple. She respected and admired Dr. Greenough and said she learned so much in his class, and that it was the best class she took for her PhD. She received her PhD in Animal Science from the University of Illinois in 1989. Her thesis centered on the effect of environmental enrichment on the behavior and central nervous systems of animals. She concluded that the brain is very plastic and responsive to stimulation from the environment.

Once again, Temple was ahead of the times. Years later, studies on brain plasticity, growth of new neural circuits, and connections in response to stimulants were rampant. Dr. Michael Merzenich, a neuroscientist from the University of California at San Francisco Medical Center, has been researching the subject. He spoke at Technology/Entertainment/Design (TED) in 2004, saying, "You can do things tomorrow that you can't do today. Individual skills and abilities are shaped by the environment, constructed from a wealth of experiences. The brain has a very powerful ability to change itself well into adulthood.

"The brain is at the mercy of the sound environment in which it is received, but the changes induced by skills are massive. What you pay attention to is why you are a specialist in your skills. Your brain is very different from the brain of someone 100 years ago and certainly 1000 years ago."

Dr. Merzenich and other neuroplasticity researchers caused quite a stir when they demonstrated that the adult brain can change in fundamental ways, like manual dexterity and perception of sounds.

For more than three decades, Dr. Merzenich has been a leading pioneer in brain plasticity research. He is founding CEO of Scientific Learning Corporation, which markets and distributes software that applies principles of brain plasticity to assist children with language learning and reading.

Dr. Merzenich uses his research to help children with autism and their malfunctioning sound systems. An excellent example of brain plasticity is Temple herself. Her language receiver in childhood was distorted and undoubtedly noisy. She has continued to grow and improve throughout her life.

CHAPTER 6

TEMPLE IN THE NINETIES

In 1991, Uta Frith translated Hans Asperger's work into English. Asperger's insights provided awareness of a broad continuum of autistic disorders. And Frith's own book (as editor), *Autism and Asperger Syndrome,* gave an account of Asperger's as a distinct variant of autism, considerably widening the concept.

"There are children and adults who can manage to pass as 'normal,' yet are fundamentally autistic," said Oliver Sacks, a professor of neurology and author. He wrote about Temple and six others in *An Anthropologist on Mars.*

Including Asperger's in *Diagnostic Manual of Mental Disorders-IV* in 1994 significantly paved the way for reframing autism as a spectrum. Asperger's quickly gained a reputation as high-functioning autism.

This new awareness of Asperger's partially paved the way for Temple's recognition. Parents, teachers, and family members were dealing with a diagnosis they knew nothing about. At autism conferences, they eagerly listened to Temple's explanations of the world from her perspective.

She reached even more people after *Thinking in Pictures* was published in 1995. She had also written an article in 1992 about the hug machine for the *Journal of Child and Adolescent Psychopharmacology.*

By now, Temple had upgraded the machine to include thick foam rubber padding and deep pressure stimulation. Users can relax fully, because the body is completely supported.

"The contoured padding provides an even pressure across the body. The foam-padded headrest and padded neck opening are covered with soft fake fur. When the neck opening closes around the neck, it enhances the feeling of being surrounded and contained by the embrace of the deep touch pressure squeeze," Temple explained.[1]

We now know that autism is caused by neurological abnormalities that shut the child off from neurotypical touching and hugging. The hug machine provides touches and hugs in a way autistics can accept without experiencing overwhelming physical sensations. It is currently used in many classrooms for autistic children.

When Temple used the machine for fifteen minutes, it reduced anxiety for up to forty-five to sixty minutes.[2] She used it twice a day for maximum effect.[3]

As Temple relaxed, her relationship with her pet changed. "The cat that used to run away from me now would stay with me, because I had learned to caress him with a gentler touch. I had to be comforted before I could give comfort to the cat." She also noticed she flinched less often when people touched her.

About the same time her article about the hug machine was published, Temple was hired as an associate professor in the department of animal science at Colorado State University in Fort Collins, Colorado. It proved a good fit. Colorado State provides a strong focus on agriculture and livestock studies for its students.

She had been there only a year when she met Mark Deesing. Mark had grown up in Salt Lake City and went to horseshoeing school because his family didn't have enough money to send him to college. He was working as a farrier to make a living and interested in getting involved in horse behavior because he had some research ideas.

A horseshoeing professor at Colorado State invited him to come and talk about horseshoeing. After his talk, a graduate student came up to him and said, "You have some provocative ideas, and I know who would be interested in hearing about them."

The graduate student and Mark walked across the street, where she introduced him to Temple. Mark and Temple clicked right away. They did research together and soon published articles in scientific journals.

Four years after they met, the owner of the building in which they worked came by to say he wanted a new facility. "I can design that," said Mark.

"Give it a shot," said Temple.

Mark did a scale drawing by hand, using the paper, pencils, and rulers Temple had advised him to use. He followed what she said, using the same tools, and produced 24-by-36-inch blueprint drawings for buildings during the next several years. By that time, engineers were using the AutoCAD program for drawings. Mark decided he wanted to work with AutoCAD.

Temple sent him to school to learn AutoCAD. Now he utilizes the program all the time. And he is currently Temple's employee.

Temple and Mark work together a great deal, often having lunch together on Saturday at one of two restaurants. He said their lunches are a combination of business and pleasure. They talk about what he's working on and what she's doing.

Mark has learned to deal with Temple's autism. "Getting to know Temple and understand her has been an experience. If she looks at you with a glazed look, there are no pictures in the pile for her, you have to find something that triggers the pack . . . People with autism focus on one subject, and go on and on with everything they know about a subject," said Mark. "You can't do a power lunch when talking about one thing."

Mark has learned to interrupt Temple when he has heard what he wants to know about the subject. "If I know what she's going to say, I just go on," he said. "People think it's rude to interrupt. Sometimes I find myself interrupting other people, especially if I know what the conversation's about. It's hard to balance my personal life and my relationship with Temple.

"It's been a learning experience. In autism, some parts of the brain don't function well; some parts overfunction. Temple pays a lot of attention to detail, and that's rubbed off on me."

Mark and Temple always manage to find levity in situations they're discussing. However, "Temple doesn't get one-liner jokes. Her humor is unique, even childlike," he said.

As Mark's friendship and work relationship with Temple grew, her influence increased among livestock producers. Cattle organizations often invited Temple to speak because she had excellent slides and visuals. Delivery of the information was important, too. Temple absorbed helpful comments from the evaluation forms that audience members filled out. She read articles about public speaking and discovered humor was frequently mentioned, so she added jokes to her lectures. "If people laughed, I kept it. If they didn't, I'd remove it and try another," she said.[4]

She was asked to edit *Livestock Handling and Transport*, a book published in 1993 by CAB International in Oxfordshire,

United Kingdom. The third edition of the same publication, which she also edited, appeared in 2007. The goal of the book was to bring together the latest research and practical information on animal handling as well as the design of facilities and transport.

Much had changed during the intervening years, including increasing awareness of animal welfare around the world, especially in South America, Asia, and India. Another important change was the development of effective auditing programs for large, corporate meat buyers such as McDonald's, Wendy's, and Burger King. The fourth edition, edited by Temple, was published in 2014.

All aspects of animal handling are covered: handling for veterinary and husbandry procedures; stress physiology; restraint methods; transport, corral, and stockyard design; handling at slaughter plants; and welfare. Animals such as cattle, sheep, pigs, deer, and poultry are discussed.

In one article about transporting cattle, Temple's co-author was Carmen Gallo from Valdivia, Chile. Both authors have observed that on overloaded trucks, there is a higher incidence of severely bruised cattle. They listed several causes of cattle truck rollovers: driver fatigue, going too fast around corners, and narrow roads with soft shoulders. South America has many gravel dirt roads that bend and wind.

Wendy Fulwider, a graduate student of Temple's, co-authored an article in *Livestock Handling and Transport* about dairy cattle. Robots that perform the duties that the farmer would regularly do are popular on smaller family dairies with about 150–200 cows, she noted. "Producers appreciated that the robot gave them the opportunity to, for example, attend their children's school events without having to plan around milking times."[5]

A second book Temple edited was *Genetics and the Behavior of Domestic Animals* in 1998, published by Academic Press. She said: "The purpose of this book is to bridge the gap between the field of behavior genetics and research on behavior published in the animal and science and veterinary literature."

Both Temple and Mark Deesing have years of practical experience with animals, but no experience in the behavior genetics laboratory. They co-authored an article on genetics and animal welfare that was included in the book.

For example, they noted: "Due to genetic selection, the ability of a chicken to gain weight has increased phenomenally. In 1923, it took 16 weeks to produce a broiler chicken. In 1993, only 6–1/2 weeks was required."[6]

Many concerns have surfaced because of genetic alterations. "When one selects for one trait, many other traits will be affected," they noted. "It is often difficult to predict which traits will be changed."[7]

Although Temple possesses extraordinary empathy for all animals, she doesn't have much feeling otherwise. Oliver Sacks, a neurologist and author, wrote about her incredible mind in *An Anthropologist on Mars* in 1995. She consistently compares her mind to a computer with many files. She can store lots of information and retrieve it at will. But like a computer, she lacks feeling. "The emotion circuit's not hooked up, that's what's wrong," she said.[8]

"I only understand simple emotions like fear, anger, happiness and sadness," she wrote in an earlier book.[9] "There is a process for using my intellect and logical decision-making for every social decision. Emotion does not guide my decision. It is pure computing."[10]

Even music does not move her, though Temple has perfect pitch. She isn't transported to a place where logic and reason and language can't go. She doesn't connect with music, usually an international language.

The same is true with nature. Temple lives in Fort Collins, Colorado, and knows the mountains are pretty, but is not inspired or comforted by their beauty. She fails to understand why others are stirred by their grandeur.

Temple knows she can't empathize with other people's feelings. She doesn't interpret the undercurrents of emotion, the smiles, the tears, the shrugs, or the frowns that most people follow automatically on the basis of experience and encounters with others.

To compensate, she has built up a library of experiences over time, videotapes in her mind, which she plays over and over again to learn how people act in different circumstances. "She had complemented her experience by constant reading, including reading of trade journals and the *Wall Street Journal*—all of which enlarged her knowledge of the species. 'It is strictly a logical process,' she explained," Oliver Sacks wrote.[11]

"All my life, I have been an observer and I've always watched from the outside," Temple herself noted.[12] "Even today I do not feel like a grownup in the realm of social relationships."[13]

She finds much more satisfaction in her work than in being social. "I can act social, but it's like being in a play," she said. When she's around people she knows, she joins in the conversation, laughs, and cracks jokes. According to Frith, routine social relationships are well within the grasp of a person with Asperger's.

Temple makes social contacts at work. "Some of the best times in my life have been working on construction projects. I can relate to people who produce tangible results," she said.[14]

Temple finds friendship, a one-on-one relationship with another person, more difficult. In *Autism and Asperger Syndrome*, Frith writes: "Asperger's Syndrome individuals . . . do not seem to possess the knack of entering and maintaining two-way personal relationships."

However, Temple has found a friend in Mark Deesing, her only employee, co-author, and research assistant. He designs facilities for ranchers and works with employee training and handling in the slaughterhouses. They both work out of their homes. Temple travels all week, every week. Their business time together is on the phone or for lunch.

"She's very routine-oriented. That will never change. She calculates down to the minute when she leaves the house to go to the airport. She always calculates time for lunch, getting her shoes shined at the airport, and the number of phone calls to return. She calls me as she's walking down the gateway to the airplane," said Mark. "She talks until they close the door. It's part of the routine."

Temple considers sexual relationships off-limits. At a TEACCH conference at the University of North Carolina in Chapel Hill, North Carolina, Temple startled Tammy Esposito, principal at Levy, a school for severely handicapped children, when she announced to a room of perhaps two hundred people: "I don't have a sex life."

Temple has never dated. "I've remained celibate because doing so helps me avoid the many complicated social situations that are too difficult for me to handle," she said. "Even today, romantic love is just not part of my life. And you know what? That's okay with me."[15]

CHAPTER 7

PROFESSOR AT COLORADO STATE UNIVERSITY

Since 1990, Temple Grandin has been a professor at Colorado State University. Just when the stirrings of concern for animal welfare were at the beginning, she landed at CSU. Temple accelerated that process remarkably. She combined engineering, construction, psychology, and animal science to help vanquish needless suffering for millions of animals.

In the process, Temple became an international success, providing worldwide media exposure to the livestock industry and issues related to animal care. She has appeared on television shows such as *20/20, 48 Hours, CNN, Larry King Live,* and *60 Minutes.* Interviews with Temple have been broadcast on National Public Radio (NPR) in the United States and similar stations in Europe. She has been featured in *People* magazine, the *New York Times, Forbes, U.S. News and World Report,* and *Time* magazine. In 2010, *Time* named her one of the one hundred most influential people in the world.

Colorado State University in the mountain town of Fort Collins serves more than thirty thousand students. Thousands have taken classes from Temple. "I can hardly believe I'm studying with Temple Grandin," said Ruth Wiowade, Temple's graduate research assistant in 2011. "She's the best in the world at what she does, a living legend."[1]

Bernard E. Rollin, PhD, one of twelve distinguished professors at Colorado State University and professor of philosophy, animal rights, and biomedical science, has known Temple since the late 1970s. He met her when she took his veterinary medical ethics course, a required part of the veterinary curriculum at CSU since 1978.

"Temple has blossomed socially since I first knew her," he said. "Then she was reluctant even to shake hands. . . . She's a precise, demanding professor and a wonderful lecturer."

He explained how she got the job at his university. "Right after she got her doctorate at Illinois, she called me and said, 'I want a job as a professor at Colorado State.'"

Rollin explained that wasn't the way it usually works. The university contacts candidates they're interested in. Temple has never waited to be asked. She said, "I like Fort Collins. It's a beautiful place. You're there and I'm not worried about how much they pay me." Those were the magic words. The university hired her to teach a few hours but worked her full-time.

"She's been a good colleague," said Rollin.

Right after Oliver Sacks's book *An Anthropologist on Mars* came out, *People* magazine called Rollin and said, "Tell me some weird stories about Temple." Rollin refused in no uncertain terms. "She's my friend and, besides, I know a lot weirder people than Temple."

Soon after the HBO movie about Temple was released, Rollin gathered a group of colleagues together. They went to the department head and said, "Temple needs tenure. It won't look good if the public finds out she doesn't have it." The department head agreed, and Temple was given tenure.

Temple values highly the impact she has on students' lives as a professor of animal science. "I'm a professor and scientist first," she said. Autism is secondary.

Jamie, a CSU junior majoring in animal and equine sciences, said that Temple's first lecture of the semester immediately helped her understand her horse better. "I now realize my horse isn't stupid at times, just reacting to something in the environment."

Stephanie, the instructor for a therapeutic riding class at Hearts and Horses in Loveland, Colorado, near Fort Collins, has also taken a class from Temple. "I loved Temple as a professor," said Stephanie. "She told jokes." Her class used *Humane Livestock Handling*, one of Temple's books with Mark Deesing, as a textbook. Temple had them draw some of the designs from the book.

Although Temple knows they will eventually use AutoCAD, she wants each student to learn to draw by hand first. She says she gets "silly mistakes like a twenty-five-foot-long gate" from those who learn on the computer.

She gives them assignments to draw their own designs meeting certain requirements. She does this to prove that they don't need a computer program to create a workable drawing. "I might get ten different drawings that all work," said Temple.[2]

Cheryl Miller has worked as Temple's administrative assistant for ten years at Colorado State University and several more when Temple hired her after Cheryl retired from CSU.

Cheryl said, "Temple is devoted to her students. She really cares about them and does lots for them. She's identified more than one student with problems and worked with that learner individually."

Temple's methods may be unorthodox, but they work. She said, "If a student submits drawings that are full of wavy, squiggly lines instead of smooth arcs, I send them to the copy shop and tell them to photocopy pages from a book using paper in all the different pastel colors until they find the shade that helps them see better."[3]

Temple uses the method discovered by Helen Irlen in 1980 to help them improve vision. She sends them to the drugstore to try on sunglasses of various colors. "I tell them, 'Don't buy what looks good. Buy what works.'"[4]

"One student with pink-tinted lenses came rushing up to me and said, 'Oh, Dr. Grandin, I got an A on my economics quiz.'"[5] That was because the PowerPoint slides stopped jiggling and she could read the numbers on the professor's graphs. Temple's insights, drawn from Helen Irlen's ideas, about ways to improve visual acuity have proven to be valuable to students.

"I always tell my students it would be stupid to flunk out of school because you're not using tan paper or because you didn't make your computer background lavender," Temple says.[6] Or because you didn't want to wear sunglasses with an unfashionable shade of pink.

If the student has out-of-state tuition and can't afford it, Temple often pays for it from her speaking fees.

Temple teaches undergraduate courses. Undergraduates and candidates for a master's or PhD are in the same classes. Those working on a graduate degree conduct research.

Temple maintains a limited number of graduate students and directs research that assists in developing systems for animal handling and the reduction of stress and losses at packing plants. She has published her research in the areas of cattle temperament, environmental enrichment of pigs, livestock behavior during handling, bull fertility, housing dairy cattle, and effective stunning methods for cattle and hogs.

I visited the Animal Science Building at CSU in the summer of 2012 to talk with Conny Flörcke, Temple's research assistant at the time. She was on the second floor in a small cubicle with sixteen graduate students in the same room. Her desk was near the printer.

"It gets very noisy when we're all here," Conny said. Since it was summer, not all the graduate students were on campus.

Cornelia Flörcke grew up near Hamelin, Germany, the town with the story about the Pied Piper, the children, and the rats. She earned her bachelor's degree in biology with its main focus on behavior and neuroscience.

She received her master's in systems biology of the brain and behavior. During the last year of her studies, she attended the Netherlands Institute of Ecology (NIOO), the top research institute of the Royal Netherlands Academy of Arts and Sciences (KNAW), located in Wageningen, Netherlands.

"Temple Grandin" was a topic in one of her lectures at the institute. Conny was fascinated by what she heard about Temple's animal behavior theories. She had always felt strongly about the livestock industry because her grandparents had a farm where she interacted with cows, pigs, and chickens, and she loved spending time with the animals.

"My grandpa was and is someone I will always look up to because he taught me so much about animal behavior and how to treat animals the right way," said Conny.

Fascinated by what she heard from the lecture, Conny visited Temple's website. She and Temple spoke on the phone in July 2009 and each talked about her research. Conny started thinking about pursuing her PhD at CSU.

Conny visited CSU and met Temple on two different days for lunch. It was important to Conny to meet Temple in person, because starting a PhD in a foreign country is difficult.

She wanted to make sure she could connect with her supervisor. They bonded quickly, and Conny noticed that Temple was already introducing her to faculty members as her new graduate research assistant.

Conny came to Colorado State to earn her PhD under Temple Grandin. "It's easy to do a dissertation under Temple," Conny said. Temple travels constantly, but makes many phone calls to Conny, making sure she knows what to do next.

"She has good advice, gives clear instructions, and listens well," Conny said. "I've gained a great deal of knowledge from her. For instance, I've become independent in my research. Part of the job as research assistant is being a teaching assistant and working with students.

"And I've picked up a lot of information about autism. I didn't know anything about autism before I met Temple. I've also learned a great deal about the livestock industry—cows, pigs, poultry."

Conny did her dissertation on cow/calf protection, including how cows that are calm may fail to protect their calves. She spent three months on a Red Angus ranch in Colorado to study how cows protect their newborn calves.

Numerous studies have shown that beef cattle selected for a calm temperament improve weight gain and meat quality. However, some ranchers comment that tame cows are not properly protecting their calves from wolves. Some ranchers' losses have exceeded twenty percent. Good protective behaviors will become increasingly important as wolves move into more and more states.

Conny made a three-minute video for *Beef* magazine in June 2012. The article, "Study Examines Cow's Protection Behavior," by Temple Grandin and Cornelia Flörcke, appeared in *Beef* magazine in June 2012.

Researching with Temple pays off. "Temple's students get great jobs," said Cheryl Miller.

Dr. Kurt Vogel, a recent student of Temple's, is on the faculty at the University of Wisconsin in River Falls, where he teaches animal welfare and animal physiology. His research interests include food, animal behavior, the ethics of animal use, and the impact of management strategies on welfare, physiology, and product quality. He receives rave reviews from his students and has earned the respect of beef journalists.

Vogel has absorbed Temple's lessons on the treatment of animals: "My point is that most of society still understands that beef and milk come from the cattle, pork comes from pigs, and chicken and eggs come from chickens. For the most part, they don't know the intricate details of how to raise and convert these animals to meat, but that is not necessarily mandatory. If they choose to consume meat, milk, and eggs, then they have a legitimate right to know how the animals are cared for if they would like to. They also have the right to ask questions about these processes. Animal agriculture has a legitimate obligation to educate, answer questions, and fix any legitimate problems that are identified by interested consumers."

Vogel was raised on a dairy farm in Wisconsin, and has always been interested in dairy cows. While working at a slaughterhouse for used-up dairy cows when he was nineteen, he developed a restrainer for the older cows, but couldn't get it to function properly. One day the general manager called him into the office. Kurt was shaking when he appeared before the GM, because he thought he was going to get fired.

"I want you to watch this DVD," said the manager. He handed Kurt a video called *Cattle Handling in Meat Plants*, with Temple's business card taped on it. "Go ahead and call my friend Temple," he said.

Kurt did. He and Temple found that they had a common ground in their interests. When he was ready for graduate school, Temple invited Kurt to work on his PhD at Colorado State.

He was a research assistant for Temple Grandin from 2008–2010. His dissertation discussed the impact of management on milk and meat. He focused on the practical and on making positive changes.

He said that Temple was a pragmatic professor. She gave vivid descriptions that were easy to picture. She was objective, not easily swayed by emotion. She called a spade a spade. And she is passionate about what she does. Because she's so intense, her students hang on to every word.

"Working with Temple was one of the highlights of my life," said Kurt. Temple and Kurt visited slaughterhouses for dairy cows past their prime. "She understands what goes on inside an animal slaughterhouse. We built a bond, sharing inside stories about experiences in an abattoir."

Although she works ceaselessly, Temple understands that people have lives outside of research. "She was respectful of my relationship with my wife," said Kurt. "She understood I wanted to have quality family time."

Another of Temple's students who grew up on a dairy farm in Wisconsin is Wendy Fulwider. Wendy has a bizarre sense of humor and has the distinction of being able to make Temple laugh. Wendy was thirty-four when she started her bachelor's degree in zoology at the University of Wisconsin, Oshkosh. She met Temple in Quebec while working on her master's in dairy management. She didn't know Temple was famous. Temple hired Wendy as a graduate teaching assistant while studying for her PhD in animal behavior. "Those were the best years of my life," said Wendy. Grandin, an inclusive professor, took her to ranches and slaughterhouses and autism conferences. Wendy wrote papers on wild animals and visited more than ninety thousand cows on 113 dairy farms in five states for her dissertation.

In 2009, Dr. Fulwider became the animal husbandry specialist for CROPP (Coulee Region Organic Produce Pool Cooperative) in La Farge, Wisconsin. She has helped more than twelve hundred beef, dairy, egg, poultry, and swine producers understand the importance of meaningful and measurable standards regarding animal husbandry and the importance of these standards as part of an Organic System Plan.

"Wendy created her own job," said Cheryl Miller.

CROPP is the nation's largest organic farmer cooperative, with a diverse product line and a varying member base. It gives organic farmers a unique opportunity to market products under their own label. CROPP sells meat products under the "Organic Prairie" label.

Organic foods represent four percent of total food sales, and it's rising every year. Consumers are demanding food produced without antibiotics, hormones, and toxic pesticides. "Temple still calls me when she has a question about something organic," said Wendy.

In 2014 Fulwider began a job as consultant for Global Animal Partnership in Oshkosh, Wisconsin.

Temple's students' jobs vary, but most of them find extraordinary employment. Her influence and ideas will survive and thrive, not only through her books and videos, but also through those who have studied under her.

PART II

AUTISM

CHAPTER 8

AUTISM ADVOCATE

Autism affects people of all races, incomes, ethnic groups, and religions. Temple speaks about people with autism every day. She's also an advocate, one who supports a cause. "Too much emphasis is being put on the deficits of autism and not enough on the strengths," she often says.

An obvious deficit is the area of social skills. Being social is not everything in life. People with Asperger's have been the doers, the inventers, the thinkers since the beginning of human development. "Some guy with high-functioning Asperger's developed the first spear. It wasn't developed by the social one yakking around the campfire," Temple said.[1]

Many of the great minds in history probably had Asperger's. "You can find examples of inventors and engineers with instinctive insights into complex problems throughout history. Perhaps they were Aspergians too," writes John Elder Robison in *Be Different: Adventures of a Free-Range Aspergian.*

Einstein was a visual thinker who failed his high school language requirement. Yet in 1999, *Time* magazine named Albert Einstein the "Man of the (Twentieth) Century." Three of his papers published in 1905 led to lasers, global positioning satellites, and the atomic bomb.

Vint Cerf, Bob Kahn, and other computer scientists who must have had Asperger's are credited with inventing the Internet. Mark Zuckerman, who created Facebook, has certain qualities of Asperger's. Steve Jobs, founder of Apple and Apple products, had Asperger's traits. The technology revolution of the twenty-first century has led to a mecca for Aspies, who feel comfortable with computers.

Jennifer McIlwee Myers, who has Asperger's, explains: "The computer's just there. It doesn't pick up on context. It doesn't care how I'm feeling. It doesn't care if my facial expression and body posture are correct. Exactly what I say, it does."[2]

Daniel Tammet, born in 1979 in England, was diagnosed with autism but went on to write *Born on a Blue Day: Inside the Extraordinary Mind of an Autistic Savant,* a best-selling memoir, and two other books. His work has been published in twenty languages. He recited pi from memory to 22,514 digits in five hours. Daniel has learned ten languages, including Romanian, Gaelic, Welch, and Icelandic, which he learned in a week. Who knows what talented people with autism will do in the future?

People with autism have several strengths, one of which is the ability to develop systems. "A system is anything that takes inputs and delivers outputs. It could be technical, like a computer, natural, like the weather, abstract, like the field of mathematics, organizable, like a DVD collection, or motoric, like a tennis shot. What is important about a system is that it is predictable and can be controlled," writes Thomas Armstrong, PhD, in *Neurodiversity: Discovering the Extraordinary Gifts of Autism, ADHD, Dyslexia, and Other Brain Differences.* Systems feel comfortable to people with Asperger's.

Another gift of autism is the ability to see details. In her book, *Animals in Translation: Using the Mysteries of Autism to Decode Animal Behavior,* Temple lists eighteen tiny details that scare farm animals, including reflections on smooth metal, metal clanging, and sudden changes in color of equipment. She has used her ability to pay attention to details in constructing equipment for animals.

Many neurotypical people consider overattention to details as a deficit. However, it can be a strength. "An individual in the Congo had all the classic signs of autism, but was regarded as gifted by his tribe. He was a master weaver. His love of meticulous detail and patterns gave him an important niche in the community," writes Thomas Armstrong.

Creativity is one more strength of autism. Temple says, "Bottom up, details-first thinkers like myself are more likely to have creative breakthroughs just because we don't know where we're going. We expect surprises. An attention to details, a hefty memory, and an ability to make associations can all work together to make the unlikely creative leap more likely."[3]

Knowing the strengths, skills, and talents of people with autism gives one more respect for those who do not function well socially.

Temple emphasizes that further exploration is needed in sensory issues, which are complex and prevalent among those on the spectrum. "A person who can't imagine being in a world of sensory overload is possibly going to underestimate the severity of someone else's sensations and the impact on that person's life, even misinterpreting behavior," she said.[4]

Having grown up with severe sensitivities in the areas of touch and hearing, Temple is very much aware of how much sensory sensitivities influence quality of life. Yet research in this area is ridiculously scant.

She wrote: "In 2001, I contributed an article to a big scholarly book on autism. More than fourteen hundred pages. Eighty-one articles in all. Guess what. The only paper that addressed sensory problems was mine."[5]

Perhaps autism researchers don't realize how pervasive the problem is. "They can't imagine a world where scratchy clothes make you feel as if you're on fire or where a siren sounds like someone is drilling a hole into my skull," Temple said.[6] Unfortunately, people differ in their sensitivities, making it extremely difficult for researchers to study. "Something that was downright painful for me could go unnoticed by someone else," says John Robison in *Be Different.*

In spite of this difficulty and the skepticism that these sensitivities even exist, someone who has lived with sensory sensitivities or someone who has loved someone with sensory sensitivities is very much aware of the reality of their existence.

"Sound sensitivity can make it impossible for some people on the spectrum to tolerate normal places such as restaurants, offices, and sports events. These extreme auditory problems can occur in both nonverbal individuals and those who are very high-functioning, like college-educated people with Asperger's," Temple explains.[7]

Sounds can interfere with eye contact, which is important to neurotypical people. According to Temple, "Eye contact is still difficult for me in noisy rooms, because it interferes with hearing. It's like my brain wiring only lets one function or the other, but depending on the circumstances, not both at the same time."[8]

If someone as mature as Temple finds eye contact in noisy rooms difficult, think about how difficult it would be for a child on the spectrum with sound sensitivities.

"What a neurotypical person feels when someone won't make eye contact may be what a person with autism feels when someone does make eye contact," writes Temple.[9] If neurotypical people were aware of this, they might better understand someone on the spectrum who doesn't make eye contact.

Any of the senses can malfunction. When my daughter Lisa was four, she screamed in fear when riding on the escalator. Since I also had one-year-old Michelle in a stroller, a trip to the mall proved challenging.

Imagine my surprise when I found out years later that Lisa had visual processing difficulties. She had trouble learning to read and was diagnosed as dyslexic. Both dyslexia and her perceptions of the escalator can be traced to visual processing difficulties.

Even when he was younger, my dad hated driving at night. He also didn't like going into dark movie theaters because of "night blindness." He had mild vision processing problems, too. A person doesn't have to be on the spectrum to have sensory issues.

Sensory disorders are not just an autism problem. Studies of nonautistic children have shown that more than half have a sensory symptom, and one in six has a sensory problem significant enough to affect his or her daily life.

"Sensory issues are very real and I think they are more a matter of degree rather than being either present or absent in people," Temple noted.[10]

Temple has participated in multiple autism conferences across the United States as well as in England, Canada, New Zealand, and Australia. She's been to France and other non-English speaking countries to talk about autism, where her speeches are translated for local audiences.

Along with writing books and speaking about her experiences at conferences, Temple advises parents of children with autism and the kids themselves at conferences and book signings.

Betty Lehman, executive director of the Autism Society of Colorado, said, "When people have children and they say, 'Maybe they'll grow up to be president,' we (parents of a child with autism) can say, 'Maybe they'll grow up to be Temple Grandin.'"

"For people on the autism spectrum and people who work in the field, this is like meeting a rock star," said Connie Erbert, an autism specialist in Wichita, Kansas. "Her story gives so much hope."

Mike Sieman of Cargill said, "I'd been to livestock conferences with Temple and she is esteemed there. But she has far more emotional impact on parents, children, and educators of those with autism."

Temple shares her life. She impacted me through her books because she explained how Jan, my autistic sister, can see and hear details others can't. "Animals and autistic people don't have to be paying attention to something in order to see it. Things like jiggly chains pop out at us. They *grab* our attention whether we want them to or not," she wrote.[11]

Temple says, "We can't filter stuff out. All the zillions and zillions of sensory details in the world come into our conscious awareness and we get overwhelmed. We're seeing, hearing, and feeling all the things no one else can."[12] Her words gave me insight into some of Jan's problems.

Temple gives tips to parents of kids on the spectrum. "The trick for parents of children with autism is distinguishing between physical problems or physical ailments and bad behavior. I was expected to sit still at the table for twenty minutes, and I did. Sometimes you have to do things you don't want to," said Temple, who believes in discipline. She benefitted a great deal from her mother's discipline.

She advises those with Asperger's on dealing with sensory problems. She encouraged a fourteen-year-old with Asperger's to "use headphones to block out unwanted sounds, just not all the time."

I was behind a mother at a book signing when I heard Temple say, "Get your four-year-old with autism at least twenty hours a week of therapy."

Temple is very practical. She knows that children need speech therapy. They also need to learn basic social skills such as taking turns; board games and card games are good instruction methods. Some of the first words they should learn are "please" and "thank you." Table manners are important, too. So is behaving appropriately in a store or restaurant and being on time. These are all skills that can and should be learned.

She complains about people who protect their Asperger's kids too much. "Get those kids out into the world!" Temple advises.

Temple suggests that you not allow your children to stay home and watch television or play video games. They need to be exposed to a variety of situations so they'll know what interests them. The world is full of fascinating and life-altering things, but kids aren't going to try them if they don't know about them.

"It's essential for an ASD [autism spectrum disorder] kid to get outside the house and accept responsibility for tasks that other people want done—and need to be done on *their* schedule. Because that's how *work* works in the real world," she writes.[13]

Kids who are eleven or twelve can play in an orchestra or mow the lawn. Playing in an orchestra is not a paying job, but it requires cooperation with others as well as a regular commitment of time. And it's doing something worthwhile that will build self-esteem.

Evan, who has Asperger's, will be a senior in high school next year. He has a summer job with a company that cleans up after a house is built. Evan has dug trenches, helped the electrician, and done some landscaping. He works forty hours a week. It's hard work and he's tired, but he likes it. And he's benefitting in many ways.

Evan doesn't like school. His mother has a hard time getting him up to go to school, but he gets himself up and off to work. He's had two raises because he's such a hard worker. At home, he's also opening up, talking more, and expressing himself within his family. His mother and grandmother have worried about him because he's so quiet and doesn't usually take the initiative in doing things. When his boss told him he needed hard-toed boots, he drove himself to the shoe store and bought himself a pair. His mother and grandmother consider that real progress.

The focus on deficits is so intense and so automatic that people lose sight of the strengths of autistic children. "Rethink the problem. I want to hear about their interests, their strengths, their hopes. I want them to have the same advantages and opportunities in education and the marketplace that I did," Temple says.[14]

What's your child's favorite subject? What does he like? What is she good at? Does he have any hobbies?

Everybody knows someone on the autism/Asperger's continuum. Temple Grandin is living proof that the characteristics of autism can be modified and controlled. Autism tends to become less extreme as the person ages and learns to cope with it better.

After all, as Jerry Newport wrote in *Your Life Is Not a Label*: "No one is completely autistic or completely neurotypical. Even God has his autistic moments, which is why the planets all spin."

CHAPTER 9

EUSTACIA CUTLER

"People who have loved a person with autism are your best resources," said Eustacia Cutler. Eustacia, mother of Temple Grandin, was one of the first to wander through unknown waters as she overcame the difficulties of challenging the system for her autistic child. She understands the myth, reality, angst, and guilt a mother experiences in coping with a child who has autism.

Nevertheless, she sympathizes with fathers. "Autism is especially difficult for men. It insults their sense of honor to father an imperfect child."

Siblings cope with a lot of negative emotions, too. I know. I'm the sibling of a person with severe autism.

I met Eustacia Cutler at an "Autism Across the Lifespan" conference given by Johnson County Community College in Overland Park, Kansas, a suburb of Kansas City. I'm sure she was surprised when I greeted her with, "I'm writing about your daughter." I explained that I grew up in the 1950s with an autistic sister, showed her the cover of my book, *A Different Kind of Kin*, and gave her a copy.

Eustacia responded with characteristic graciousness. After her keynote speech, I saw her several times throughout the day, spoke to her at lunch, and even caught her dozing in the last session when we were all tired.

Now in her eighties, a small, perky woman with curly hair, Eustacia has four children, three younger than Temple. She lectures nationally and internationally on autism. She earned a B.A. from Harvard after her divorce, was a band singer at the Pierre Hotel in New York, and performed and composed music for the cabaret.

Her current book, *A Thorn in My Pocket*, describes raising Temple in the conservative world of the 1950s when children with autism were automatically institutionalized.

Eustacia notes that children on the autism spectrum are literal and have trouble understanding what they cannot see or touch. She says these children have difficulties with conceptual thinking (understanding the idea of something), context (the place we're in and the situation), eye contact (understanding messages received this way), and shared information (understanding that the mind of someone else is separate and different from my own).

But she readily points out that these children can learn and grow. "We're the only species born with an open skull," she says. "Genes are far from being fixed."

Temple has proved that. She has succeeded beyond Eustacia's wildest dreams. "The older I get, the less autistic I am," said Temple. She interacts with so many neurotypicals that she's had to change. "If you call the boss an asshole, he won't give you a job," she notes.

Scientists have long suspected that the brain of an autistic is different from the brain of a neurotypical. Autism may be caused by disruption in connective circuits in the brain. On October 3, 2011, Temple had a brain scan on CBS's *60 Minutes* to show that she really does have a different kind of mind. Leslie Stahl, a broadcast journalist, and Dr. Walter Schneider, a neuroscientist from the University of Pennsylvania, looked at the results on national television, comparing Temple's brain with one of a neurotypical person.

"There's a dramatic difference," Leslie said.

The neuroscientist agreed. Fibers in the neurotypical brain were tight and organized. Fibers in Temple's brain were all over the place, a dramatic disorganization of wiring.

"Of course, we'll have to scan more autistic brains to know for sure," said Dr. Schneider, "but someday neurologists may be able to diagnose autism by scanning the brain."

Eustacia recommends the work of V. S. Ramachandran, a medical bioneurological researcher named by *Newsweek* as one of the most important people to watch in the twenty-first century, to her audiences—parents and teachers of those with autism. Ramachandran said, "the uniquely human sense of self is not an airy nothing: without habitation and a name . . . the self actually emerges from a reciprocity of interactions with others . . ." Since people with autism have trouble interacting with others and interpreting those interactions, no wonder their sense of self is so shaky!

Ramachandran wrote *Phantoms in the Brain: Probing the Mysteries of the Human Mind,* a fascinating book. He says, "Freud's most valuable contribution was his discovery that your conscious mind is simply a façade and that you are completely unaware of ninety percent of what really goes on in your brain."[1]

Temple claims not to have an unconscious mind. She does not repress memories and thoughts like neurotypical people.

"There are no files in my memory that are repressed. You have files that are blocked. I have none so painful that they are blocked. The amygdala locks the files of the hippocampus. In me, the amygdala doesn't generate enough emotion to unlock the files of the hippocampus," she wrote.[2] Every visual impression of the world around her remains accessible in her conscious mind. One of the corollaries of possessing a powerful and detailed visual memory and not possessing an unconscious is that Grandin has no place to repress her memories.

"Denial's an emotion I don't have," she said. "I don't understand denial."[3]

Ben Cutler, Temple's stepfather, was an orchestra leader whose sounds ushered the society set from swing to rock to disco and back again. He worked in all the right places in New York, from the Persian Room at the Plaza to the roof of the Astor Hotel. He taught himself to play the soprano saxophone.

Eustacia and Ben had been married for thirty-six years when Ben died on January 5, 2001 in Bronxville, New York, at the age of ninety-six. By then Eustacia was well-established on the speaking circuit. She had officially started speaking to groups in 1999 when Wayne Gilpin, the president of Future Horizons, which publishes many books about autism and organizes conferences about it, asked her to make a trip to England to speak to mothers of children with autism. As the number of children with autism has increased, so has the need for information.

Many in the audience at conferences have a newly diagnosed child. The whole family echoes the confusion. "When the usual responses can't grow, consciously and unconsciously, a whole family is changed," Eustacia writes.[4]

In 1951, Eustacia must have felt alone in a world where autism was virtually unknown and only diagnosed in one of every ten thousand. She was fortunate to have money and to have Dr. Caruthers, who recommended that Temple have an EEG to see if she had petit mal, a mild form of epilepsy.

"The autism/epilepsy connection wouldn't be discovered for another fifteen years, which puts Dr. Caruthers neurologically way ahead of his time," Eustacia wrote.[5] He was the expert who also recommended speech therapy and nursery school for Temple.

Eustacia came up with the idea of a nanny herself.

Eustacia continued following her remarkable instincts. "I was prepared for the workforce from an early age," said Temple. "I had an alarm clock to get me up in first grade. At age thirteen, I worked for a dressmaker for an afternoon every week. In high school, I shingled a shed. People with Asperger's need to learn to do things."

To encourage her interest in art, Temple's mother bought her daughter professional art materials and a book on perspective art drawing when she was in grade school. Like most mothers in the 1950s, Eustacia insisted on good behavior. By the age of five, Temple had to dress up and behave in church and sit through formal dinners at home and at her grandmother's house.[6]

Eustacia did not let Temple lie around the house and never viewed her daughter's autism as rendering her incapable.[7] She was a good detective about what environments caused Temple stress. She recognized that large crowds and too much commotion were more than Temple's nervous system could handle. When Temple had a tantrum, Eustacia usually understood why.[8]

When Temple was very young, Eustacia allowed her one hour every day after lunch to revert to autistic behaviors. During that hour Temple had to stay in her room. "Sometimes

I spent the entire hour spinning a decorative brass plate that covered a bolt that held my bed frame together. I would spin it at different speeds and was fascinated at how different speeds affected the number of times the brass plate spun," Temple recalled.[9]

With her extraordinary insights into her child's needs and her instincts for finding ways to improve her child's life, Eustacia Grandin is a good role model for mothers who have a child with autism.

CHAPTER 10

NORM LEDGIN

I met Norm Ledgin at a Kansas Authors Club Conference in Lawrence, Kansas. Norm and I both belong to KAC. His district was taking its turn hosting the state conference. I appeared alone in the breakfast shop at the hotel and looked for someone to sit with. I spotted Norm sitting by himself. Knowing he had written *Diagnosing Jefferson* and *Asperger's and Self-Esteem*, and aware we have a common interest in autism, I asked if he minded if I sat with him. He responded graciously.

After we'd talked for a while, I said, "I'd like to write about Temple Grandin."

"What do you want to know?" Norm asked. "I know her well. When you're ready to call her, let me know and I'll give you her number." We kept in contact after the conference.

After I'd done a lot of research and writing about Temple, he said, "It's time to call her. Let me give you Temple's number." He did. I nervously called and left my phone number. In about two hours, Temple responded. Since then, I've communicated with her numerous times.

After speaking with both Norm and Temple, I realized that their worlds collided. Temple says she takes satisfaction from realizing she has "something in common with a Founding Father." She and Thomas Jefferson are both on the autism–Asperger continuum, which Norm Ledgin pointed out.

Norm Ledgin published *Diagnosing Jefferson: Evidence of a Condition That Guided His Beliefs, Behavior, and Personal Associations* in 2000, which identified Thomas Jefferson's Asperger's characteristics.

Norm and his wife Marsha are the parents of two children, one of whom has Asperger's. Their son Fred received the diagnosis only two years after Asperger's was defined in the *Diagnostic and Statistical Manual of Mental Disorders*. He was diagnosed in 1996 after his parents had consulted psychologists, psychiatrists, education counselors, learning disabilities specialists, and others for nine years. The psychologist who made the diagnosis handed Ledgin an article on Asperger's. That was the first time the Ledgins had ever heard of or read about the condition. A school district staffer, who knew Fred had been diagnosed with Asperger's, recommended Ledgin attend a conference in Chicago. Fred and his father both attended. They heard Temple speak, but they found little information there on Asperger's.

This is not surprising considering Hans Asperger's paper was only translated into English in 1991. Asperger, an Austrian pediatrician, published a paper in 1944 that described the characteristics of a milder, high-functioning form of autism. Asperger's takes its name from him.

Ledgin's interest in Jefferson goes back to high school, when he realized Jefferson was essentially a liberal philosopher, though many of his beliefs formed a basis for conservative views as well. At the time he decided to write about Jefferson, Ledgin was reading one biography after another and was in the midst of the six-volume work by Dumas Malone.

Ledgin writes, "Moving through major biographies about him over a period of several years, I concluded by the summer of 1998 that the repeated mentioning of his various idiosyncrasies suggested a pattern of behavior begging for identification. I noticed Jefferson's biographers reached points in their narratives where they were forced to offer rationalizations for his oddities before moving on."[1]

Ledgin had observed that his son Fred's view of reality appeared different from most other people's views, and he started tracking Fred's Asperger's condition. This led him again to Jefferson. He followed the similarities between Fred and Jefferson, and at first found twenty. When he found fifty, he started writing a manuscript, which he showed to Temple Grandin. She pored over three drafts before agreeing that Ledgin had made his point credibly. "Her patience with me was unlimited, and there was a driving force to her enthusiasm," Ledgin wrote.[2] "We talked on the phone mostly and actually met face to face at conferences in Kansas City and Denver in the late nineties."[3] Ledgin also drove to Denver to hear Tony Attwood, an Australian psychologist and author of several acclaimed books on Asperger's.

Later, Ledgin realized there were other achievers in history with whom he could match modern diagnostic criteria for Asperger's syndrome. That led to his lecturing on the subject of role models and, eventually, to writing *Asperger's and Self-Esteem*. He researched biographies of famous geniuses to find that Asperger's often contributed to their success.

In this book, Ledgin included Albert Einstein, Charles Darwin, Orson Welles, Oscar Levant, Marie Curie, Paul Robeson, Gregor Mendel, Béla Bartók, Carl Sagan, Glenn Gould, John Hartford, and Wolfgang Amadeus Mozart.

His books have opened readers' eyes to the positive side of Asperger's. Parents thank him for turning around the lives of their diagnosed children. He gives them hope in a world where the youngsters had felt like aliens.

Ledgin says: "I knew that my positive views would be useful, perhaps inspiring to parents of Asperger's youngsters and especially to the teens themselves. Instead of making the kid feel strange, *the parent can make him or her feel proud of who he or she is.* It's a pretty big deal to be in the company of Jefferson, Einstein, and Mozart. And there's certainly no shame in being different as respect grows for the benefits of diversity."

Although no two people with Asperger's are exactly alike, Ledgin benefitted from his son, Fred. He saw firsthand "literalness, routinization, perhaps too strict an adherence to rules, a surprising use of advanced logic, a dogged pursuit of details, a hammering away at fixations, and a few uncommon perspectives of humor."[4]

Diane Kennedy, an author and advocate for Asperger's syndrome, writes: "They are our visionaries, scientists, diplomats, inventers, artists, writers, and musicians. They are the original thinkers and a driving force in our culture."

Many adults are now being diagnosed with Asperger's. Scotty, diagnosed with Asperger's at twenty-four, says: "What do Batman, umbrellas, Marilyn Monroe, and retired pharmaceuticals of the 1950s have in common? I have been obsessed with all of them over the years." Adults with Asperger's need to know all about topics that grab their attention.

Susan Boyle, the singer, was diagnosed with Asperger's at age fifty-two. She said she felt relieved. "I have always known that I had an unfair label put on me," she said in the interview with the *Observer* newspaper. The church volunteer from a small Scottish town became a global sensation when she sang "I Dreamed a Dream" from *Les Misérables* on *Britain's Got Talent* in 2009.

The contrast between her shy manner and soaring voice won Boyle legions of fans. She has sold more than fourteen million records around the world. The singer said she was glad she and others would now have a better understanding of the struggles she has experienced.

One of the reasons people think those with Asperger's are peculiar is because of their sensory issues. Although these are not specifically mentioned as a criteria for diagnosis, they should be. "Some adults with Asperger's consider their sensory sensitivity [to have] a greater impact on their daily lives than problems with making friends, managing emotions, and finding appropriate employment," according to the *Complete Guide to Asperger's.*

Ledgin remains an advocate for those diagnosed with Asperger's. He still speaks at area conferences on the subject. He teaches a course in continuing education at the University of Kansas titled, "Explaining the Perplexing Thomas Jefferson," the core of which is the condition to which Ledgin attributes Jefferson's range of idiosyncrasies as well as his talents.

"I may be the first writer to come out and say that some of our geniuses made significant contributions creatively because of Asperger's syndrome," Ledgin said. "That's because I know people with Asperger's think differently from the way the rest of us think. The fact that so many of these contributions are unique leads me to believe we wouldn't have had the benefit of them without the Asperger's condition."

CHAPTER 11

CONNIE ERBERT

Connie Erbert has spent her career working with children and adults challenged by autism, especially Asperger's. According to the Centers for Disease Control and Prevention (CDC), one of every 68 eight-year-olds is diagnosed with autism in the United States. There are plenty of opportunities.

In 2007, when Connie Erbert came to Heartspring, a world-renowned institution in Wichita, Kansas, for persons with disabilities, she started the first Asperger's day camp in Kansas, called Social Skills Technology Asperger's Recreation Camp (SSTAR). Kids came to SSTAR from all over Kansas. I volunteered to help.

The campers—ages three to twenty-one—were divided into groups by age. Since Asperger's is more common among boys, there were lots more boys than girls. The group just older than ours, filled with students from second through fifth grade, included only one girl.

Our group worked on social skills. At first, the students just sat there while teachers and assistants attempted to interact with the participants. We divided into two groups and threw marshmallows at one another. We again divided into two groups and wrapped colorful crepe paper around two of the students to create animals. In the beginning, I played many games of Connect Four with Clark, one of the campers. Gradually, the students made friends with each other.

Not that there weren't problems. Brian had a huge meltdown the second day. Connie, a tall, powerful woman, carried him out of the room kicking and screaming. People scurried out of the way. Helpers moved several chairs. Connie called his mother to come and get him. He was back the next day, and he was fine.

At the end of the week when I arrived a little late, I was amazed at what I heard. The kids played together quietly in groups of two or three, obviously getting along. They had finally found a place they could fit in, some for the first time.

"Connie is our Mary Poppins," said Teri Loper, the parent of a child on the spectrum, who spoke at a ceremony honoring Connie. "She offers answers, guidance, understanding, patience, and love. Like Mary Poppins, Connie's bag is bottomless; she continues to pull from it new and creative ideas to help those in the CARE [Community of Autism and Resources Education] program."

"I have a lot of respect for these parents," said Connie. "They live every day with the triumphs and challenges of autism. Their dedication and drive to seek out and access the appropriate resources and support for their children often puts them in positions of frustration and despair. When we are all able to find a common ground and work together for their children, it becomes a rewarding experience with a much brighter outcome."

Parents need information on how to advocate for their child. Many parents don't know how to work with the system, especially after elementary school. They need to know how to advocate for their middle schoolers or high schoolers or college age kids. Connie helps them do this.

Erbert, along with Heartspring, founded CARE in Wichita, Kansas, a metropolitan area of about 500,000 people. Assuming the statistic that one in sixty-eight people have autism is correct, there are thousands in the Wichita area with some form of autism. Through the CARE program, parents and children attend workshops, camps, and conferences specifically designed for families that have a person on the spectrum. She trains community members and business and law enforcement agencies about living with, employing, and understanding persons with autism. Every day she advocates for people on the spectrum.

For her work, Connie has received national recognition. *Exceptional Parent Magazine* honored Connie with its Model of Excellence in Education in 2008. In 2011, she received one of three Unsung Heroes of Autism awards from premium Swiss chocolatier Lindt USA and Autism Speaks.

Erbert graduated from Fort Hays State University and has done graduate work through the University of Kansas and the University of North Carolina. She worked in the Wichita public school system as the autism behavioral consultant for ten years. Erbert has presented on various topics related to autism spectrum disorders throughout the state, as well as nationally. Her training certifications in various areas of autism research include extensive, up-to-date work with the structured teaching model through the University of North Carolina TEACCH training in functional behavior analysis, assessment, and behavior intervention plans covering all aspects of developmental disabilities through the University of Florida; completion of training with the developmental, individual difference, relationship-based approach floor time model under Stanley

Greenspan and Serena Weider; training in the area of applied behavior analysis; and participation in over a hundred conferences, workshops, and symposiums throughout the United States.

Connie has spoken at the same conference as Temple Grandin many times. After a convention, she shared these observations: "Having seen Temple speak a number of times over the years, I noticed a rather substantial change in her presentation skills as well as the content of her presentation. She was much more animated [and] personable, and was able to elaborate and expand her presentation through anecdotal side stories, which made it all the more interesting. Obviously, the passage of time along with practice via her numerous speeches over the years have afforded Temple the vehicle with which to hone her lecturing skills. *A good example of how individuals with autism learn to cope as they get older.*

"I think sometimes we might forget, because autism isn't always a disability we can see, it can be a very subtle disability that sometimes becomes more evident when sensory issues crop up. In the midst of Temple's talk, and shortly after she explained her sensitivity to loud, high-pitched sounds, a door alarm was accidentally set off by one of the conference participants. It took about ten seconds for the alarm to stop, and all the while, looking at Temple's face, you could see that it was indeed painful. Barely audible was Temple's verbal response to a question she asked herself, 'Why is a burglar alarm going off in the middle of my talk?' The alarm ceased and she proceeded without even addressing the painful interruption. It was apparent she had developed coping skills for just such occasions. While the interruption was painful, she was able to get through her presentation without displaying the obvious level of discomfort she must have been feeling."

Connie was born in Mt. Clemons, Michigan, a suburb of Detroit. Since her father was in the army, her family moved frequently. When she was three, the family moved to Pueblo, Colorado. In Pueblo, she had her first memories of watching television shows, including *Mayberry RFD*. The theme of that show, which she said is "Do the right thing," stuck with her. "My job is to increase autism awareness," she said. "Increasing autism awareness increases opportunities"—opportunities for those with autism, for family members of persons with autism, and for the community. Her favorite quote is from Robert Breault: "Sometimes to do the right thing, we must keep a promise we never made."

When she started the Autism Awareness Walk in 2008 at Heartspring, she hoped people on the spectrum and their families would connect with their community in a common goal. Every year since then, the number of participants has doubled.

Connie started Camp SSTAR because she realized the need for many children with Asperger's to experience social interaction in a safe, organized, and fun environment. She also did it because those with Asperger's have so much difficulty making friends. Camp SSTAR has evolved over the years. A new greenhouse, an arts program, and new technology programs are featured. One advantage of Camp SSTAR is that Connie gets acquainted with the campers' parents and has a chance to follow up with them.

SSTAR scouts grew out of Camp SSTAR. The kids learn social skills through scouting. Also they have fun. And Connie has another chance to meet parents.

"A primary focus of my job is working with parents," she said. "I believe in the 'airplane theory': put an oxygen mask on the parent first, and then put one on the child."

She advises and informs parents. She knows they often go through difficult times. Gretchen and Sean DiGiovanni have triplet boys, Sam, Paul, and Jack. Sam has autism. Gretchen eloquently expresses the feelings of many parents: "This holiday season, while you are shopping, dining out with friends, taking kids to a Christmas activity, going to a sporting event, visiting family, entertaining in your home, exercising, or reading a book, I ask you to put yourself in the shoes of someone whose family is affected by autism. These things are challenging for them. The battle of emotions, stress, guilt, worry, and mental distress can be overwhelming and exhausting. *And* the families live with this twenty-four hours a day, seven days a week. What if he gets up in the middle of the night and gets out of the house? Why does going through the drive-thru have to be an all-out war? How are the siblings learning coping behaviors in this crazy environment? Screaming, self-injury, and inability to communicate are continuous struggles for some."[1]

As an educational consultant, Connie works with many young adults on the spectrum, including some belatedly diagnosed with Asperger's. One of those is Scotty, now twenty-four. He has struggled to come to terms with his past experiences and new diagnoses, which is painful and exhausting for him and his family. Scotty writes: "Though I had no problem plowing through the works of James Joyce entirely of my own accord, I rarely turned in my homework. I could not learn to drive or even throw a baseball. I didn't seem to understand the difference between making friends and taking hostages."

David Finch, author of *The Journal of Best Practices: A Memoir of Marriage, Asperger Syndrome, and One Man's Quest to Be a Better Husband,* told strangers at a party that he wanted to become close friends with them "as soon as possible." This speaks eloquently of the disconnect and loneliness of these often isolated persons.

Connie informs the public in a number of ways. For example, she gives talks about autism to policemen, since "a person on the spectrum is seven times more likely to have contact with the police than someone who isn't on the spectrum." Because of this, parents of young adults with autism are eager for law enforcement officials to be educated about their concerns.

When asked, she teaches local business owners. A business owner in Wichita, Jerry Winkler, asked Connie to talk to his staff about autism because his adult son, Jonathan, would be working in the family business. She talked to employees about Jonathan's talents and challenges, encouraging them to speak to him and cheer him on throughout the day. "Their understanding and willingness to learn was exemplary," she said.

Connie's class, Exploring Careers, instructs young adults with autism. They explore various options. One student toured Red Rock Canyon Grill with the restaurant's head chef as part of his career exploration. Another pulled bulbs at Botanica Gardens.

This remarkable woman receives email and phone calls from parents and clients in the area daily. As I interviewed her, the phone rang several times. "I can't talk right now, but I do want to discuss this," she said. "Give me your phone number and I'll call you tomorrow." Connie has been known to answer a call from a frantic parent in the middle of the night.

In one year, CARE staff provided many individual, family, and school consultations. With phone consultations, that number rose. Most of the meetings were within Kansas, while some were throughout the United States, and some were international. Using technology, out-of-state and international interviews were made via email or Skype.

Heartspring participates in World Reach, an organization that is dedicated to touching lives all over the world through professional training and meetings. It takes part in international conferences and collaborates with individuals and organizations in other countries.

Several from Heartspring, including Connie, traveled to China and India to train other teachers about autism. Teachers from China and India have also traveled to Heartspring.

By raising awareness and supporting families, Connie impacts lives around the world. "The more we share and care about those around us, the more we can learn, grow, and become one community of people passionate about changing the lives of those diagnosed with an autism spectrum disorder," she said.

"What works for one child doesn't necessarily work for another. You have to be flexible and try things," said Connie. "Never give up. You just don't know what will work."

Autism is a relatively new diagnosis. A cause for the majority of children with autism hasn't been found, but that's not the main focus. The issues of the individual need to be addressed, so the child can live as independently, productively, and happily as possible.

Because the cause and cure remain largely unknown, desperate parents are vulnerable to "snake oil." I have talked to family members convinced that expensive vitamins are going to cure their child of autism. Connie helps families identify strategies that will work for them.

In April 2014, Heartspring celebrated a historic Care Walk. Jonathan, a young adult with autism and a beautiful voice, sang the national anthem. Jeff Colyer, lieutenant governor of Kansas, presented a ceremonial copy of the recently passed autism insurance bill in Kansas. Connie said the bill was a "long-sought-after first step in providing increased early intervention of autism for families in Kansas." Heartspring is a good model for other places in the US.

Autism is the fastest growing underfunded developmental disability in the United States. One in every sixty-eight children has been diagnosed with autism spectrum disorder, according to the CDC. Treatment for a child with autism averages $7,000 to $9,000 a year. CARE provides services for over five hundred families a year. Nearly 60 percent seek financial assistance. No one is turned away.

The Autism CARE Walk at Heartspring is growing. In 2012, eight hundred people walked. In 2013, twenty-five hundred people walked. In 2014 almost four thousand people participated and raised $101,012. In 2016, over seven thousand people walked.

- Erbert left Heartspring in early 2015 because she saw a gap in the system for young adults with autism. An estimated fifty thousand Americans with autism will turn eighteen as part of the surge of children diagnosed in the 1990s. Many of these children have graduated from high school with average to above-average GPAs. Some have even graduated from college. Often these persons with high-functioning autism lack the social skills to acquire the employment they need to live on their own. An example is Josh Zimmerman. He graduated from college with honors, but the only job he could find was cleaning out dog cages for a veterinary clinic. He is one of many in the same situation.

- Autism Avenue Flower and Gift Shoppe opened in December 2015. It provides a structured work environment with on-the-job training and real-world work experience for young adults with high-functioning autism. It's a for-profit shop, sponsored by Independent Living Resource Center.

- The first group consisted of twenty-five individuals. The goal is for each one to live independently and obtain his or her job of choice. As individuals graduate from the program, others with similar needs will be brought in. The goal is for employees to leave Autism Avenue and enter the community workforce equipped with skills and confidence. Efforts reach far beyond the store as founders of Autism Avenue strive to educate other potential employees.

"The more we inform ourselves about autism spectrum disorders, the more we can support, encourage, and include individuals on the spectrum in our schools, workplaces, and communities," said Connie.

Fortunately, there are more and more Connies getting involved in the autism community.

CHAPTER 12

STEVE JOBS AND THREE REMARKABLE AUTISTICS

Though never formally diagnosed, Steve Jobs had many Asperger's traits. Whether the topic was computers, stock options, or pancreatic cancer, Jobs liked to make his own rules. He could focus intently, and he insisted on being in control. Unaware of people's feelings, Jobs frequently stomped on them. Brutally honest, he lacked the filter that restrains people from venting wounding thoughts. He saw things in black and white. He obsessed over details. He always dressed in a black turtleneck and jeans, even wearing the same brand. All of these traits are signs of Asperger's.

A genius, Steve Jobs will be remembered for creating the gadgets that have pervaded our lives, putting a thousand songs in our pockets, developing a microcomputer, and enabling the nonverbal to communicate. He founded a company at the intersections of art and technology, humanities and science, creativity and engineering. He possessed the greatest designer's eye in the world.

Jobs created the iPod, the iPhone, and the iPad. His Pixar entertainment company gave us *Toy Story, The Incredibles, Finding Nemo, Cars,* and *Up,* establishing the computer-generated animated feature. Credited with popularizing the computer mouse and all the Mac computers, great and small, Jobs was a giant in the world of technology.

This visionary understood he was making media. He transformed lives with the idea that computers are something that belong in your life, not a science lab. "They are not just for numbers, but also for music, movies, magazines, creation, communication. You want to use them, play with them, touch them, carry them with you," Jobs said.[1]

Steven Paul Jobs was born in San Francisco on February 24, 1955, to University of Wisconsin graduate students Abdulfattah "John" Jandali, a Syrian immigrant, and Joanne Carole Schieble. They were twenty-three. Unwed at the time, they put him up for adoption.

John and Joanne married in December 1955. Steve's sister, novelist Mona Simpson, was born in 1957. John and Joanne divorced in 1962.

Steve was adopted by Paul and Clara Jobs. When Steve was five years old, the family moved to Mountain View, California. Paul Jobs, a machinist for a company that made lasers, taught his son basic electronics and how to work with his hands. "Jobs's father taught him that a drive for perfection meant caring about the craftsmanship even of parts unseen," reports Walter Isaacson in *Steve Jobs*.[2] Though he had a better life with the Jobs family than he would have had with his biological parents, all his life Steve was haunted by his adoption.

Jobs attended junior high and high school in Cupertino, California. He frequently attended after-school lectures at Hewlett-Packard, and was later hired there. He grew up in Silicon Valley, with its mixture of engineering and counterculture.

Steve Wozniak, five years older, was an electronics hacker when he met Steve Jobs and they became friends. "Woz" made a blue box that let users make free long-distance phone calls. Jobs marketed it—their first collaboration. Ironically, much later Jobs would sue Google for selling the Android, saying they had stolen the idea from the iPhone.

After high school graduation in 1972, Jobs enrolled at Reed College, dropping out after only one semester. In 1974, he took a job as a technician at Atari, a manufacturer of video games. He saved his money for a spiritual retreat to India and came back a Buddhist with his head shaved and wearing traditional Indian clothing. He remained a Buddhist all his life. He loved the Buddhist saying: "The journey is the reward." During this period, Jobs experimented with psychedelics, which he said influenced him greatly.

At the time, his hygiene was a problem. According to Walter Isaacson, he insisted that his vegan diets meant that he didn't need to use a deodorant or take regular showers. He would soak his feet in the toilet.[3] For understandable reasons, this repulsed his co-workers. He embraced extreme diets, including purges, fasts, and eating only one or two foods, such as carrots or apples. At one point, Jobs ate so many carrots he turned orange.

The two Steves, Jobs and Wozniak, launched the Apple company out of Jobs's parents' garage in 1976. "I was nowhere near the engineer Woz was," Jobs freely admitted. "He was always the better designer."

On May 17, 1978, when Jobs was twenty-three, the same age his parents were when he was born, his daughter, Lisa Nicole, was born. Her mother was Chrisann Brennan, his first serious girlfriend. Though already wealthy, he denied paternity, while Lisa's mother went on welfare. He eventually acknowledged he was the father.

Jobs met Laurene Powell, blonde, brainy, and beautiful, while speaking at Stanford University. Laurene had graduated from Stanford with an MBA. They married on March 18, 1991. She was tough and a sensible anchor for his life.

Reed Paul Jobs was born in 1991. He adored his father and they had a great relationship. Though Reed looked like his father, he possessed attributes lacking in Steve, expressing affection and empathy. Like his dad, his favorite way of discussing a serious subject was taking a long walk.

With his daughters, Jobs was more distant. Erin Sienna was born in 1995 and Eve in 1998. The family lived in Palo Alto in an ordinary, easily accessible house.

Their half-sister, Lisa Brennan-Jobs, also lived with them off and on. Her relationship with Jobs remained rocky, though she came to visit him when he was very sick, which pleased him greatly.

On January, 24, 1984, at Apple's annual shareholders' meeting, Jobs introduced the Macintosh, which became the first commercially successful small computer with a graphical user interface. Also that year, Steve and his biological sister, Mona Simpson, found each other and became close.

At the end of 1984, the computer industry experienced a sales slump. Apple's declining sales resulted in short tempers and great tension within the company. A power struggle developed between John Sculley, Apple's CEO, and Jobs. The board of directors sided with Sculley and ousted Jobs in 1985.

Jobs remained the largest Apple stockholder with more than $85 million in shares. In 1986, he bought the Graphics Group (later renamed Pixar) from Lucasfilm's computer graphics division for $10 million.

In 1997, Jobs returned to Apple, which had acquired his new company NeXT for $400 million plus the services of Jobs.

When he came back, he was a far better manager. He revived Apple, then near bankruptcy. He became permanent CEO from 2000 until August 2011, shortly before his death. Jobs created irresistible products and great companies. Two of the best companies in his era, Apple and Pixar, were founded by Jobs.

Jobs's tumor was discovered in 2003. It turned out to be a rare and operable form of pancreatic cancer. Jobs put off surgery while searching for an alternative, which included his usual extreme diets and fasts. He waited more than nine months before having surgery and then claimed it was a success. This was a sign of his "reality distortion field," well known at Apple.

Jobs spent a lot of time building his legacy. He pushed people to perfection, inspiring loyalty to Apple. "He made me do things I didn't think I could," said one executive. He left a strong team. Jobs had taken medical leave three times, leaving Tim Cook in charge. The company performed well with Cook at the head. In August 2011, Jobs resigned from Apple.

The world watched Jobs's health anxiously, which must have been agony for Jobs, who was a very private person. He grew noticeably thinner and weaker. "His pancreas had been partly removed and his liver had been replaced, so his digestive system was faulty and had trouble absorbing protein. Losing weight made it harder to embark on aggressive drug therapies. His emaciated condition also made him more susceptible to infections," Isaacson says.[4]

He died on October 5, 2011 at the age of fifty-six. His wife Laurene, all four of his children, and his sister Mona were at his side. He had asked to be buried near Paul and Clara Jobs.

Jobs's final triumph was the Apple iPad, released in January 2009. The first month Apple sold one million iPads, which made it the most successful product chronicled in history. By

July 2011, 500,000 applications (apps) had been created. There were more than fifteen billion downloads.

"What Jobs did was perfect other people's inventions. He optimized them. He buffed and polished other people's ideas. Jobs wasn't an idea man; he was a remix artist," says journalist Lev Grossman.[5]

Jobs understood what the public wanted and even anticipated it, transforming several industries in his lifetime. His life can be summarized by a commercial Apple made in 1997, which included the line: "The people who are crazy enough to think they can change the world are the ones who do."

The iPad helped a group in which Jobs had little interest: nonverbal autistics, which represent approximately 30 percent of persons with autism. Many family members and workers of those with severe autism use the iPad to communicate. Autistics like order and control, and are fascinated by the iPad. It doesn't work for everyone, but family members and workers using iPads are discovering there's more inside the heads of those with nonverbal autism than they had previously been able to express. Family members and workers had suspected this for years.

What's new about the iPads is that it's a mainstream device being used for communication with the nonverbal. The iPad is far less expensive than most other speech communication devices, and it's easy to carry.

Temple Grandin said, "Unlike computers, in tablets the keyboard is actually part of the screen, so eye movement from keyboard to the letter being typed is minimal. Cause and effect have a much higher correlation. That difference could well be meaningful in allowing people with extreme sensory problems to communicate."[6]

"The speed at which this has taken off and become entwined in special education is something I've never seen before," said Lindsay Dutton, MA, CCC-SLP, director of School Therapy and Applied Technology at Heartspring.

At Heartspring, autistic children undergo an extensive evaluation to see what kind of communication device and which apps or programs are best for them. Children are tested on six to eight different devices. "There are a lot of communication devices. We want to find the right fit for the student, not fit tech to students, so we test on a variety of devices. We don't try to fit the iPod or iPad to the student," said Dutton.

In order to get insurance to pay for the device, a qualified speech therapist has to do the AAC (Augmentative Alternative Communication) evaluation. If the communication tool is an iPad, there are numerous apps available. The apps vary in quality. "People writing apps don't necessarily have a language background," said Dutton.

"There's no peer-reviewed research on iPads; it's all anecdotal," said Dutton. "There's a newness factor that parents should be aware of." However, some children benefit enormously.

The Grace app gives some nonverbal autistics a chance to "speak" for the first time. It starts with four hundred images that were chosen by nonverbal people as communication starters. Categories include colors, food and drink, my body, and places. *Grace* allows the users to build their "photo vocabulary" by snapping their own photos to use within the app. The app's creator, Lisa Domican, named *Grace* after her autistic daughter.

Another app is *iConverse*, five communication tiles that represent basic needs: food, drink, bathroom break, sick, and help.

An AAC (Alternative Augmentative Communication) device can be as simple as making gestures to interact. And you don't have to be nonverbal to benefit from it.

These tools allow a child to express their feelings, thoughts, and needs. He can ask for things at home and school. She can be understood better with less frustration. The goal is to encourage independent social interaction by allowing the child to take control.

* * *

Soma Mukhopadyay from Bangalore, India, developed a method that parents of autistic children are really excited about. Her son, Tito, is severely autistic with uncontrollable movements, but he writes eloquently and independently about his autism and what it is like. His poetry reminds us that you cannot assume what is going on inside the head of someone who is unable to communicate.

When Tito failed to develop properly, Soma, a former chemistry teacher, took him to doctors in India. She ignored their warnings about her son's lack of abilities. From infancy, she read constantly to him. She watched Tito stare at a calendar, wanting to understand it. When he was two and a half, she started teaching him to count and read the alphabet, using a chart. Soma read Tito one of Aesop's fables and asked him what it was about. He pointed to letters on the chart that spelled out "crow." Assuming he understood, she read to her son from Dickens, Hardy, and Shakespeare. She educated him in mathematics, including geometry. She played classical music. All this time, Tito was in constant motion of tremors and paroxysms, eyes gazing far off. Soma ignored this.

She moved his limbs through the motions Tito needed to make in order to write, helping him feel the muscle movements, talking all the time. She attached a pencil to his right hand with elastic bands and guided him as he traced the alphabet on paper. This tireless and tenacious taskmaster prodded her son constantly, still talking. At the age of six, he began to write by himself using a pencil.

From eight to eleven, Tito and his mother wrote *The Mind Tree: A Miraculous Child Breaks the Silence of Autism,* an accumulation of heartfelt and startling perceptions about being imprisoned inside an autistic body and mind.

Tito remembers looking at himself in a mirror, willing his mouth to move. "The image stared back," he wrote. This only emphasized the third-person point of view that disconnected his thinking self and his acting self.

Now Tito and his mother are in the United States, astounding people in the autism world. They are an outstanding example of what parents may be able to teach their children.

An interviewer asked Tito, "What would your life be like if your mother had not taught you?" He wrote: "I would be a vegetable."

Dr. Michael Merzenich is emeritus professor from the University of California at San Francisco Medical Center. Dr. Merzenich has a BS from the University of Portland and a PhD from Johns Hopkins. He's a well-known neuroscientist who specializes in brain plasticity, the brain's ability to change.

"That's probably a fair assessment," Dr. Merzenich said, confirming what Tito would have been like if his mother hadn't worked with him. "He's a beautiful example of the possible," he said.

Soma has used effective, noninvasive tools to bring children with autism out of their shells. She is now the educational director of Helping Autism through Learning and Outreach (HALO). She developed the Rapid Prompting Method (RPM) to teach her son. Soma educates people with autism on how to learn and reason, how to communicate and express ideas. She shows people with autism, previously unreachable, how to let people in and how to know who they are.

Soma emphasized her no-nonsense approach in an interview on Danaroc.com. "Just because Tito has autism doesn't stop me from insisting he pick up his clothes and clean his room just like everyone else.

"Everyone participates in society. I'm short, but I am still a part of society. Tito has autism, but he's still one of us. An autistic child just needs someone to do certain things for him. Everybody needs something. *We all need each other.*

"If you sit over there and expect and hope, you are wasting good energy," added Soma.

* * *

Jeremy was born in 1989 and shortly afterward diagnosed as severely autistic. When he started high school, he was in a class for severely mentally handicapped students. In 2010, Jeremy graduated from Torrey Pines High School in San Diego with a 3.7 grade point average. At his high school graduation, he gave one of the commencement speeches.

Jeremy was fourteen when he went to Soma Mukhopadyay. His mother, Chantal Sicile-Kira, who lives in San Diego, drove Jeremy to Los Angeles, two hours each way, to see Soma twice a month for a year and a half. Soma taught Chantal as well as Jeremy.

Jeremy and his mother wrote a book together called *A Full Life with Autism: From Learning to Forming Relationships to*

Achieving Independence. A former TV producer based in France, Chantal is an award-winning author, columnist, and speaker on autism.

Though he obviously thinks, Jeremy remains essentially nonverbal. He has written articles for publication and wants to be a writer who explains what it's like to have autism. Jeremy wrote, "Having autism hinders my ability to talk, not my ability to think."

Jeremy communicates several ways. He has some verbal requests and points to written words and phrases. He uses a QWERTY keyboard as a letter board. His high-tech communication devices include an iPad or Lightwriter (a portable text to speech communication aid).

Chantal knew all the therapies available and had the resources to try them. Jeremy has benefitted greatly. One of Jeremy's many difficulties is auditory processing problems. After Auditory Integration Therapy (AIT), he said, "Before therapy, I heard all sounds the same. I could not pick out the voice of the person speaking to me from the sounds in the background. I believed all sounds were noise."[7]

He has received treatment for vision processing problems as well. Jeremy said, "Before vision therapy, I could only see fragments instead of seeing objects as a whole. Faces looked like portraits painted by Picasso."[8] Jeremy has benefitted greatly from his therapy.

* * *

Naoki Higashida was born in Japan in 1992. He wrote *The Reason I Jump: The Inner Voice of a Thirteen-Year-Old Boy with Autism* with David Mitchell. This slim book in question-and-answer format was published in Japan in 2007 and in the US in 2013. It became a *New York Times* best-seller.

Naoki said, "Many children with autism don't have the means to express themselves and often even their own parents don't have a clue what they may be thinking."[9] Naoki wrote this because, thanks to his mother and an excellent teacher, he can express himself. He also had access to David Mitchell, who has a child with autism, and his wife, Ka Yoshida, who translated Naoki's book from Japanese.

Naoki answers many questions about why people with autism do what they do. For instance: Why do people with autism talk so loudly and weirdly? He said, "When I'm talking in a weird voice, I'm not doing it on purpose. I'd be okay with a weird voice on my own, but I'm aware that it bothers other people."[10]

Until recently, no one knew how to reach the thousands of nonverbal autistics, each trapped in his own world. Many have not had the advantages that Jeremy and Tito had. Of course, there are different levels of intelligence among people with autism as there are among all people. Still, many more must be reachable.

CHAPTER 13

TWO SEVERE AUTISTICS

"**A**utistic children seem 'wild' for a lot of different reasons," Temple explains. "A huge problem for autistic children is scrambled processing. The world isn't coming in right. So young autistic children end up looking wild for the same reason Helen Keller looked wild: parents and teachers can't get through to them."[1]

The families of Jan (my sister) and Neil (who we will discuss later in this chapter) include older children who had developed normally, so their parents knew what normal development was like. I'm sure neither set of parents knew anything about "scrambled processing." My sister Jan was born in 1954. Our parents had never known anybody like her. Neil was born in 1994. He had four older neurotypical siblings. His parents were baffled, too.

"Autistic people have so much natural fear and anxiety that when they're young they can be like little wild animals. For years people thought autistic people were unreachable because they were uncontrollable. A lot of people think that the feral children we've heard about over the years were actually autistic," said Temple.[2]

We certainly knew about the "wild" part. Jan was large for her age, wiry, wiggly, and fast. She had blonde braids, brown eyes, and olive skin, tanned from her beloved outdoors. Mama, who only weighed 110 pounds, said, "Jan was always going in every direction, except the one she was supposed to. I knew I had to have my running shoes on to keep up with her."

At that time, we had no understanding of the topsy-turvy world she lived in. We did know Jan had autism. But even that much knowledge was rare for that time and place. We lived on a farm in Kansas. Jan had been diagnosed in Chicago in 1958 when she was four years old. We and most of the rest of the world had no idea what autism meant. Leo Kanner had discovered it only eleven years before Jan's birth.

According to Temple, a high fever at a young age is one of the causes of autism. Jan experienced a high fever at the age of eight and a half months. Though we didn't know it at the time, Jan probably had encephalitis.

Temple also says that autism is caused by "a complex inheritance of many interacting factors." There are often milder traits in siblings, parents, and other close relatives. Some traits that seem to be associated with autism are intellectual giftedness, shyness, learning disabilities, depression, anxiety, and alcoholism.[3]

Many of our relatives displayed one or more of these traits. Jan was the only one with autism.

Jan recovered slowly from her fever, able only to drink 7Up for a couple weeks after her illness. For many days she was pale and weak. Soon after she recovered, we noticed a change in her personality. "Jan stopped talking and concentrated on walking," my mother wrote in her baby book.

And walk she did. This active, into-everything child disregarded personal harm. She crawled on top of whatever she could reach, ran into the street, and disappeared when no one was watching her. Then the tantrums started—screaming and throwing herself on the floor when crossed or sometimes for no reason. By the age of eighteen months, she said nothing with meaning. Her conniption fits and contrary ways began to dominate our family life.

One Sunday in church, I watched Mama as she tried to get Jan to cooperate and then watched our neighbor as she dealt with her fifteen-month-old twin boys in the next pew. "Jan's more trouble than Joan Wilson's twins," I whispered.

Jan's behavior only worsened with time. She ignored the world around her, not answering requests and ignoring orders. She mixed sugar and cigarette ashes on the kitchen table and then danced a jig on top of it, just to make sure it spread everywhere. Sometimes she threw things on the floor, seeming to delight in the sounds they made. It was almost impossible to know what would make her laugh or dance with glee. She disregarded horrified reactions.

We took her to family gatherings, but she showed no interest in being part of the group. Mama or Daddy had to stay with her constantly. Even then, temper tantrums were frequent and unpredictable. Daddy stayed with her while the rest of us attended church.

Much later in the teacher's lounge when I was teaching, I described some of Jan's behavior. A self-righteous teacher said, "I wouldn't have allowed it."

Sure, I thought, knowing she had one well-behaved daughter. My mother's first two children behaved well. Mama, shocked by Jan's antics, didn't have the knowledge or training to stop them. She had Jan all day, every day, with nobody except Daddy to relieve her. No schooling was available for severe autistics in the 1950s.

There were many things I didn't understand about my little sister. I recall Jan running into the kitchen, grabbing a spoon, and racing out again to the back steps. Then she tossed it up on the roof of the back porch, dancing and giggling. She did this over and over again, with spoons and spatulas. When too many utensils collected on the roof, Mama sent Bruce, my younger brother, through the tiny bathroom window to retrieve them.

Jan refused to sit with us at meals. For a long time she ate peas, but eventually she would only eat peanut butter and honey sandwiches. My mother mixed vitamins and medication into the peanut butter, then left a peanut butter sandwich and a cup of milk on the corner of the kitchen table. Jan drank a great deal of milk, frequently dumping what she didn't want on the floor.

She rocked in her shabby rocking chair incessantly. Her recurring tantrums were ear-splitting and lengthy. She flung herself on the floor and kicked her heels for no reason that we could comprehend. Sometimes she knocked her head on the floor or the back of her rocking chair as she rocked. Life with Jan was a blur of activity and unpredictability, overwhelming for us all.

Often Mama called Bruce to calm her. He put his arms around her tightly until she could control herself. "No one was closer to Jan than Bruce," said Mama.

We were fortunate that the Institute of Logopedics in Wichita, Kansas, a national and international leader in the treatment of speech disorders, was only sixty-five miles from us. The unfortunate part was that Mama had to drive with Jan twice a week to the institute for speech therapy. Each time Mama asked somebody (usually a great-aunt) to accompany them. Mama was terrified of the traffic in the city.

One day when nobody was with them, they got a flat tire. Mama knew she had to change it. It would be minutes, even hours, before someone would come along to help. She got out of the car, telling Jan to stay in the car, and changed the tire. When she returned to the car to get back in, Jan had locked all the doors and was laughing inside. Fortunately, since she had just used the key to unlock the trunk, she had it in her hand. Otherwise, she did not know how she would have solved this dilemma on a lonely road.

Only two weeks later, Dad was driving our family down the road, Jan at his side, rocking contentedly. Suddenly, she reached over, grabbed the key, and tossed it out the open window.

"She threw the key out!" he yelled. He pulled the car over to the side of the road. Mama stayed with Jan. The rest of us searched in the weeds along the roadside. No key. Because of the way the car was made, it could run without a key after it was started. He drove back to the house where a spare key waited. For the rest of his driving days, Daddy carried a spare key in his billfold.

Keeping clothes on Jan required constant vigilance. We lived in the country and visitors arrived infrequently, so most of the time we didn't bother. When Jan was very young, she bolted out of the house naked and danced on top of the car. Daddy protested. He thought she would make dents in the top of the car. Little did he know what a problem it would become.

As Jan grew older, she kept up her nude dancing on top of our vehicle. Both my parents had many other responsibilities and no help with Jan. Though watching Jan was a high priority, it was impossible to keep track of her every second.

Daddy was on the school board in our small school district. Getting good teachers was a problem. He interviewed potential candidates in the front yard. One time when he was interviewing a prospective teacher, a naked Jan, then about six, burst out of the house without clothes on, climbed on top of our car, and frolicked. We found out what had happened when Daddy roared into the house holding Jan's hand. I seldom saw him that angry. "Great balls of fire!" he hollered, red-faced with anger. The teacher did not take the job.

I have no idea why Jan danced on top of the car. I do have some thoughts about why she took her clothes off. According to Temple Grandin in *Autistic Brain,* taking clothes off is a sign of tactile sensitivity. Even today, Temple says: "Clothing drives me crazy if it's not the right texture." She cannot stand some cotton T-shirts because they're too scratchy, even if they've been washed.

Some people with autism are famous for breaking glass. Jan broke her share. She stepped through a window pane under which my mother was growing small plants. Blood streamed from her foot. We rushed her to the emergency room where she received over a hundred stitches.

Her milk cup was plastic. We learned not to leave glasses where she could reach them, but at that time milk came in glass gallon jugs. Jan managed to break many of them. She stuck her foot through window panes. Daddy patched them with cardboard until he could get a replacement.

Glass shatters and scatters incredible distances. Tiny pieces could be found across the room. Mama learned that a wet paper towel picks up most of the shards. At the age of sixty, I still shudder at the sound of breaking glass.

When Jan was seven, our baby brother, Lee Robert, was born. I enjoyed him immensely, and felt even diapering was not a chore. When Lee was six months, Jan grabbed a large, sharp-edged shovel in the yard and threw it at him. Fortunately, she missed, but my parents were concerned about the consequences of Lee and Jan living in the same house. They decided Jan had to be institutionalized.

Jan was evaluated at Kansas Neurological Institute. I remember waiting in the lobby with Bruce and Lee for a long time. A tall, skinny man in a brown suit with a notepad watched us intently for a while. Then he disappeared. After waiting for what seemed like an eternity, Mama and Daddy and Jan reappeared. Mama told me later the man who observed us was a psychologist. "He told me anyone who'd been living with Jan should have therapy," she said.

Mama and Daddy had to break the news to Jan that she was going to be institutionalized. They told her she was going to school.

Inevitably, the day came when she had to leave. "Goin' to 'cool, goin' to 'cool," she sang over and over, until she realized it was too far for her to come home at night. Then she reared back her head, hitting Mama in the face. Mama had a black eye for weeks.

A month later, we made the four-hour drive to visit her. When Jan climbed into her accustomed spot between our parents, I hardly recognized her. She was pale, thin, and neatly groomed. Her blonde braids had been chopped off and her hair clung to her head. We took her to a park where she could swing, but mostly we drove around. She rocked back and forth in the front seat.

When we returned to the cottage, I again held Lee while Mama and Daddy took Jan inside. They were gone a long time. When they came back, Mama opened the car door, climbed in and burst into tears. "They said she's hardly eaten since she's been here," Mama said. "She just sits in her chair and rocks." Daddy started the car and we began the journey home.

My sister Carol was born on December 11, 1964. Mama took Carol to a photographer for her six-month picture. "Look how much Carol resembles Jan," she said.

That summer Jan came home from the institution for her regular visit. She behaved abominably, even more than usual. Possibly, she resented this new intruder. On some level, Jan knew she'd been cheated. We continued to visit her at the institution, but she never came home again.

As Jan approached adolescence, she, like one-third of all persons with autism, developed seizures. Hers were violent and frequent. For a while her social worker called regularly to report how many seizures she'd had that week and informed my parents about medication changes. At least once during this period when they took a group to the zoo, Jan went in a wheelchair. I found it hard to picture my formerly fleet little sister confined to a wheelchair.

Jan died in a van accident on a field trip with members of her cottage. She was forty. Her death was as unexpected as her life.

* * *

According to Temple, "The landscape I was born into sixty-five years ago was a very different place from where we are now. We've gone from institutionalizing children with severe autism to trying to provide them the most fulfilling lives possible."[4]

Born in 1994, Neil Carney is the youngest of five. His siblings, Zach, Kathleen, Martin, and Tim, are all neurotypical. Neil was diagnosed with severe autism at the age of three. His family have been through a great deal. His parents, Aldona and Pat, support each other. Pat was one of eleven children, one of whom was disabled.

Aldona and Pat are proactive in getting services for their child. They speak up because they know that there are many families who can relate to what they are going through. They also know there are vulnerable, nonverbal people who have no one to advocate for them, which they will always do for Neil.

Neil requires round-the-clock, one-on-one care. He is part of a subset of people with autism who are violent. His family desperately needs help. People have no idea what the Carneys go through just to take a family outing.

Aldona and Pat wrote this in a letter to the editor in the *Wichita Eagle:*

1. Have you ever had a doctor tell you that your child has a lifelong disability with no known cure?
2. Have you ever cleaned up feces that were smeared all over the room or changed a thirteen-year-old's Pull-Up?
3. Have you ever had to fight off attacks from an adult child while he was in a rage? Or watch, horrified, as he pulls out his own adult tooth?
4. Have you ever had to stop your child from attacking other people while in public? Or had to take turns going to church?
5. Have you ever had to stay up most of the night for many nights in a row because your child doesn't have a normal sleep cycle, but still be expected to perform at your job?
6. Have you ever had to have poison control on speed dial because your child eats or drinks inedible things?
7. Have you ever had your heart ripped out because you had to leave your child at a state institution so

he could be safely detoxed off an antipsychotic drug
that was no longer effective?

Neil is a flight risk and he is fascinated with water. Once, the
school system lost him for an hour. There was an all-out search,
including a helicopter overhead. They found him in a ditch by
some water. He was moved to Levy, a school for the severely,
multiple handicapped, where the security was much tighter.

Besides severe autism, Neil has been diagnosed with MR
(mental retardation), ADHD (attention deficit hyperactiv-
ity disorder), OCD (obsessive compulsive disorder), and pica
(eats inedible things). He has consumed three baby mattresses.
He can't be exposed to light bulbs because he has attempted to
eat them. He has swallowed insulation and charcoal.

He will eat too much of a food he likes. Neil doesn't have
a shut-off valve that stops him from eating. He will eat until
he throws up. Now, Neil lives in an extended family teaching
home (EFT) where there are locks on all the cabinets.

From the time he was a baby, Neil was different from his
siblings. He only slept in a baby swing. He loved the motion.
He stopped nursing at four months. All the other kids had
nursed for a year.

When he was two, Rainbows (a school for preschool devel-
opmentally disabled children) diagnosed him as developmen-
tally delayed. The Carneys took Neil to Valarie Kerschen, MD,
a developmental specialist in Wichita, who diagnosed him at
three and a half with severe autism and profound retardation.

"I thought it would get easier as he got older," said Aldona,
"but it got progressively harder." At eight years old, Neil still
wasn't sleeping through the night, so Dr. Kerschen started him
on a low dose of Seroquel to help him sleep. It worked for
a while, but eventually lost its effectiveness, so Dr. Kerschen
upped the dosage. This continued for a number of years.

Besides not sleeping, Neil was very difficult to potty train. He had a habit of smearing feces all over his room. When he was finally potty trained at thirteen, the family had a celebration, but that wasn't his only issue.

When puberty kicked in, Neil became much more aggressive. Gradually, the Seroquel lost its effectiveness. He ripped apart clothing. He bit his older brother deeply enough to send him to the emergency room.

At seventeen, Neil experienced intense violent rages. He attacked Aldona and other caregivers. Once in a fit of rage, he sank his teeth into the carpet and pulled out his own adult tooth, root and all. His brother, Martin, who stands six-foot-five inches, was able to manhandle Neil.

"I can't give Neil any more medication. It's not working anyway. He needs to be removed from the home and detoxed," said Dr. Kerschen.

Both Aldona and Dr. Kerschen called multiple places to find a psychiatric facility that would take Neil. They heard many no's. He needed one-on-one round-the-clock supervision. "We just don't have the manpower to take him," they heard repeatedly.

Finally, Parsons State Hospital admitted him. He took his glider rocking chair with him to Parsons. He was there for a year. Aldona and Pat visited him often. Neil also rode a bus that brought him to Wichita, where someone in the family picked him up. When he came home, he was totally off the drug, although it probably took two to three years to clear his system.

Neil received a Money Follows Person (MFP) federal grant that helps people transition out of institutional living. To receive the grant, the person has to have lived in an institution or psychiatric residential care facility for at least ninety days. The money can be used for the transition items needed to move and the safety and medical needs of the person moving into the community.

Pat and Aldona bought a HUD home with the help of two of Pat's brothers and totally remodeled it. They fixed it up specifically for Neil's needs. A humidifier on the furnace because of his eczema. No exposed light bulbs because of his pica. Shut-off valves on the hot water heater because of his attraction to water. They completed the fence in his backyard because he is a flight risk. This is the EFT house.

Neil has a teacher, Bethany, who lives with him. Neil loves Bethany. She works with him on things like washing his hands and waving good-bye, both of which have taken him years to learn.

Someone is always with Neil. The house has a bedroom for Neil, a bedroom for Bethany, a living area, and a sensory room. There are cameras in the house, monitored constantly by Community Living Opportunities (CLO) in Lawrence, Kansas. If Neil tries to leave the house, someone from CLO calls, alerting Bethany.

Because he is nineteen, he's still in school at Levy, where he will remain until he turns twenty-one, when he ages out of the school system.

Neil calls the EFT his "house." On weekends he goes to his "home," where he grew up.

"I have the same goal for all my kids," said Aldona. "I want them to be happy, healthy, and as independent as possible."

Aldona has given many speeches to the legislature advocating for those with autism. "She's always giving a speech somewhere," said her son Tim.

Because Neil's behavior deteriorates when he has tooth problems, Aldona advocated for dental care for persons with developmental disabilities. "Now there are some dentists in Wichita who will take persons with special needs," she said.

Aldona was a physical education teacher for many years. "I always did a unit on autism during April, autism awareness month. Many parents called and said thank you for informing us.

"Autism is a huge spectrum. Some kids are very noisy with lots of body-rocking and hand-flapping. Education is the key. It's tolerated so much better now."

"Would I change Neil?" asked Aldona. "Yes, I would change the autism. The stress is huge and constant. There's always something. You have to have a sense of humor.

"Some people say, 'God won't give you any more than you can handle.' I'm with Mother Teresa, who said, 'I just wish he didn't trust me so much.'"

PART III

ANIMALS FOR FOOD

CHAPTER 14

CREEKSTONE FARMS: THE MODEL SLAUGHTERHOUSE

I was going to visit Creekstone Farms Premium Beef Packing Plant in Arkansas City, Kansas, primarily because Temple Grandin had designed the facility. I had an interview with Jim Rogers, director of marketing.

"You're going to get to see Creekstone," Temple said. "It's a beautiful facility."

I enjoyed the drive—tall sunflowers with large golden heads crowded many of the ditches. I passed a pecan grove, small towns I knew by name only, and stands hawking homegrown produce. I saw some green crops, but also many fields full of weeds or brown corn stalks, dried up from lack of rain.

Creekstone is north of Arkansas City beneath the city water tower, but no GPS was going to tell me that. I found it after asking directions.

I finally located the entrance to the plant, marked with a welcome sign for visitors. A multitude of glass doors look out over the parking lot. Creekstone's $185 million, 450,000-square-foot packing plant was built in 2001. When I visited, it was still one of the most advanced slaughterhouses in the country. It employed seven hundred people, important to the economy of Arkansas City, a town of 11,000 people.

After a short wait in the reception area, Jim bounded down the stairs to meet me. He's almost a foot taller and at least twenty years younger than I am. We introduced ourselves and he led me to his office. A *New York Times* article heralding Creekstone Farms beef was on the wall. It held a multitude of plaques from places where their products are sold. I knew Creekstone sold beef to many high-profile restaurants in New York, but there are many others.

"What do you want to see?" Jim asked.

"Everything," I replied.

"Even where a cow is stunned?"

"Yes," I said, "but ask me again when we get there."

"I will," he said.

We walked a short distance before we suited up, a requirement by health and safety regulations. We wore jackets, hairnets under our hats, and white gloves. He handed me earplugs and booties to slip over my shoes. The journey began.

In the first area, workers were grinding up beef for hamburger. The beef came from cattle that had been tested for *E. coli* and mad cow disease and only from those raised in certain pastures by farmers approved by Creekstone Beef.

We moved to the carving area. First, each carcass is opened at the twelfth rib, exposing the rib-eye and revealing the marbling. A grader from the United States Department of Agriculture examined the carcasses. Wielding their sharpened knives, butchers carved some nine hundred carcasses swinging on computerized trolleys, riding rail after rail as they were cut up. One of the workers constantly sprayed water.

Jim said, "We discharge into the Arkansas River approximately 600,000 gallons of water daily. This water has been treated by our on-site water treatment plant and is as clean or cleaner than the water already in the Arkansas River."

I noticed the smell was much less offensive than the packing plant in Emporia, Kansas, where I'd gone to college in the 1970s. One reason is that Creekstone processes fewer animals. In an industry that processes more than 600,000 head of cattle weekly, Creekstone, with its 5,000 head a week, accounts for less than 1 percent of the total number of animals. Fewer cattle helps reduce the stench.

Another reason for less stench is the airflow. "Our facility has separate air handling units for each department. There it circulates to our harvest department [dirtier part of the plant]. It does not mix with air in our fabrication department [cleaner part of the plant], which helps reduce the risk of contamination," Jim said.

Workers labeled every piece of meat and then entered the number into the computer. Later, if there was a problem, it could be tracked for future reference.

We climbed the stairs, holding on to the railing as the sign cautioned. I spotted several small pieces of stray meat tracked in by worker's shoes on the stairway. In the packing area, workers sealed meat in cold bags and packed it in dry ice for shipping. Boxes were stacked high.

"The innards section will be warm and smelly," Jim warned. It was, though not nearly as smelly as I expected. I easily identified the liver and the heart.

He showed me the black tongues of Angus cows. "In Japan, black tongues are a delicacy," he said. "We ship our tongues to Japan."

We moved to the area where workers stripped black hides. Black hides hung in various stages of stripping. I knew *E. coli* is often found in the skins. "All cattle have *E. coli*," said

Jim. "Cattle don't care where they lie. They frequently lie in manure."

I was especially interested in the next part, which Temple Grandin had designed. "In 2000, Creekstone gave Dr. Grandin a pencil and piece of paper and told her not to worry about money," said Jim. At the time, it was owned by a company called Future Beef. Creekstone is the result.

By then, Temple was esteemed in the livestock business. Her methods of advocating humane treatment for animals had proven successful. Benefits of humane treatment are both gratifying and profitable. She says calm handling practices reduce the animals' fear and stress. Treating animals humanely decreases injuries both to animals and their handlers.

Grandin uses natural behavior to keep cattle comfortable. I saw how cows followed each other up the ramp to slaughter. I recalled my dad holding open the gate for the lead cow. Then we watched as cows, steers, and calves trailed across the road, one after another, to the other pasture.

Jim and I walked above the pens. Each pen held twenty-eight animals. Black faces and an occasional white one, which meant a Hereford had slipped in somewhere, looked up calmly. The silence awed me. I grew up on a farm, but had never been around this many perfectly quiet cows.

"Mooing means stress," Jim said. I remembered an example of stressed-out cows and calves in my childhood when the dam of a neighbor's pond broke because of excess rain. We lived half a mile away, but that night was filled with constant mooing as the cows struggled to cope with unexpected water.

At Creekstone, silent cows follow each other to the stun area. When Jim and I were there, workers from the stun area were on break, so I didn't get to see a cow knocked out. I was disappointed because I knew how important fast and painless stunning has been to Temple.

I did get to see the center-track restraining system Temple invented. It's been installed in half the slaughterhouses in North America. The restraining system is a conveyor belt that goes under the animal's chest and belly. The animals straddle it lengthwise the same way they would straddle a sawhorse.

Temple said, "The reason plants have adopted my design is that animals are much more willing to walk onto it than they are the old V-shaped restraining systems, so it's a lot more efficient."[1]

Temple has thought a lot about this. "I was upset that I had just designed a really efficient slaughter plant. Cows are the animals I love best."[2]

She decided that she can live with her slaughterhouse designs because we need cows for food. She has been very influential in giving cows a decent death. Cattle slaughter can be calm, efficient, and humane. At one plant, "Each fat steer walked onto the conveyer belt and settled down like a little old lady getting on a bus," Temple wrote.[3] Most of the cows received a pat on the behind as they got on. Since they were close to their buddies, they weren't at all afraid.

Grandin said, "I used to wonder if the animals knew they were going to be slaughtered. I watched them going into the squeeze chute on the feedlot, getting their shots, and going up the ramp at a slaughter plant. No difference. If they knew they were going to die, you'd see much more agitated behavior."[4]

After my trip to Creekstone, my husband Dave and I visited Chester's Chophouse and Wine Bar in Wichita, which uses beef from Creekstone. This was a fancier restaurant than we usually patronize, but the service was excellent and we both found the food marvelous. "It was expensive, but we'll go back," Dave said. "It's been years since I had a steak so delicious."

CHAPTER 15

IMPROVING ANIMAL WELFARE

Because he knows Temple Grandin, I had asked for an interview with Dr. Mike Siemen, head of Cargill's animal welfare, which is based in Wichita. I parked on the street beside Cargill's new Innovation Center, a just-opened $15 million, 75,000-square-foot building. I entered the building and the receptionist looked Siemen up on the computer while I signed in and filled out a name tag.

Dr. Siemen appeared before I was finished. We introduced ourselves and rode the elevator to the fifth floor, winding through a multitude of cubes to his office.

On the wall was a poster of Claire Danes, the actress who played Temple in the award-winning docudrama, *Temple Grandin*. Next to it was a large photo of the real Temple, dressed in her customary western wear.

Cargill, an international producer and marketer of food and agricultural, financial, and industrial products and services, employs 130,000 people in sixty-three countries. The company has had a close working relationship with Temple.

When founded in 1865 in Minnesota by W. W. Cargill, they made a large grain elevator. Today the company has agricultural projects in many countries, including China, Russia, France, and Canada. They have many elevators storing wheat in the United States.

The company has recently opened research centers around the world, but this is the only one for the company's meat operations. Cargill Meat Solutions is an umbrella for seven companies involved in pork, beef, and poultry processing, marketing, and distribution. Cargill Beef is the largest of the units.

As Connie Erbert of Heartspring had predicted, Mike Siemen was easy to talk to. He'd been with Cargill for five years and worked with Temple for twenty-five. "We think a lot of her," he said. "Her ideas make sense and they work. She's persuasive and credible. She understands livestock and has greatly improved facilities. No one could have forecast Temple, born in Boston, would be a livestock expert."

Temple flies all over the world, speaking to groups and talking to officials at livestock facilities and meatpacking plants. Her calendar is full for the next two years. "She keeps it in pencil, so she can erase easily," said Siemen. "She's in the air every other day."

He had changed the time of our original appointment because he needed to videotape Temple. When checking with Temple, she had two hours for taping in San Antonio on Friday. "She needs plenty of time on both ends for videotaping to be productive," said Siemen. "She doesn't like to be stressed when getting on flights. When Temple said, 'I'm done at noon and don't fly out until seven o'clock ,' that was perfect. She doesn't have that much time again for a month." Consequently, our interview was on August 29, which happened to be Temple's birthday.

Where livestock are concerned, Temple's sensory skills are tuned in. "She focuses on things differently. She hones in on things faster," said Siemen, which is "an advantage to her in this industry."

I already knew that throughout her career, Temple has worked to improve the welfare of animals. I had read *Humane Livestock Handling: Understanding Livestock Behavior and Building Facilities for Healthier Animals*, which Temple wrote with Mark Deesing. I had also watched the video *Cattle Handling in Meat Plants*, produced by Grandin Livestock. The principle behind her designs is to use natural behavior to encourage cattle to move willingly through the system. Animals like to see where they're going. As I know from growing up on a farm, walking single file is the nature of cattle. Temple observed that cattle are calmer when they can touch each other or occasionally receive a pat on the rear end.

It isn't the habit for animals to hurry. "Let them go at their own pace," Temple said. "Calm animals are easier to handle than frightened, agitated ones." That's important, because a cow weighs 1,400 pounds or more.

"Animal handlers are often injured when frightened, agitated cattle run over them. The expense of paying hospital bills and other workmen's compensation claims or replacing employees costs the meat industry thousands of dollars each year," Temple wrote.[1]

Not only is humane handling safer for workers, it produces better meat. Every bruise directly affects meat quality. "Old bruises cause localized areas of tough meat. Fresh bruises at the meat plant cause huge losses because the bruised meat must be cut out and discarded," Temple explained.[2] "The hide does not have to be damaged to have a bruise underneath. An animal can have a huge bruise under a hide that has completely normal hair and no sign of injury."[3]

Humane handling also reduces illness in animals. "Producers who raise organic or natural beef, pork, lamb, and other meats know that keeping animals healthy is essential. Sick animals that have been treated with antibiotics cannot be sold in the organic market."[4]

Grandin's innovations don't have to be complicated or expensive. Many breakthroughs aren't. She's banned the use of electric prods. She's physically taken the electric prod out of some workers' hands, sometimes leaving the hand still moving. She calls this the "automatic prod reflex." She substitutes blue, cone-shaped plastic rattles or an inflated trash bag tied to the end of a stick for the electric prod.

She's pointed out details that disturb cattle: shadows, coats on the fences, a coffee cup on the ground, and moving people or vehicles. "They're much more afraid of a dangling chain than death," Temple said. She encourages getting down and looking at what the animals see.

Neurotypical people truly think differently than animals or autistic people. Typical people are good at seeing the big picture, but bad at seeing all the tiny details that go into that picture. Most people have brains that are structured to filter out all the tiny details that go into that picture. "The price human beings pay for having such big, fat frontal lobes," Grandin writes, "is that normal people become oblivious in a way that animals and autistic people aren't. Normal people stop seeing the details and only see the big picture."[5]

Neurotypical people are surprised when they realize how much Temple sees, but Temple has been amazed by how much ordinary people fail to see.

"The number one mistake livestock handlers make is too many cattle in the crowding pen," said Temple. The crowding pen is where they wait before slaughter. She recommends moving cattle in small bunches. "One of the most common mistakes when handling cattle and pigs is overloading the crowd pen leading to a single-file race or loading ramp. The pen should be *half* full so that the animals will have room to turn."[6]

Temple designed facilities catering to the cows' needs. Cows follow each other through the narrow passage, enjoying being near each other, and are calmed by the subdued lighting. Curved walls eliminate sharp corners (Temple's been known to put cardboard over a sharp corner until it could be changed) and blind turns that make them nervous.

Temple can look at a system and see animals walking through it. Even after the design is finished, plant managers call her to look at their plans before they change things. "Sometimes Temple will say, 'Let's make modifications.' It's cheaper to consult with Temple than to remove concrete and then pour more," said Siemen.

Two of Temple's biggest areas of concern are slaughter and the need for nonslip flooring. Cattle are much more secure if they don't feel like they're going to slip when walking. She recommends grooves in the floor where cattle are walking. "If they're not deep enough, rent a grooving machine and make them deeper," she says.

"Nonslip flooring is essential for good animal handling," she writes. " Important places to have nonslip flooring: single-file race, truck floors, veterinary facilities, stun boxes, and the crush. Small repeated slips where one hoof moves back and forth rapidly are really scary for animals."[7]

Temple is not against slaughter. She realizes the cattle were grown for food. She just wants it to be humane. Sledgehammers to knock cows out were banned in 1958 by the Humane Slaughter Act. All meat plants that sell meat to the U.S. are covered by this act. It requires that cattle, pigs, sheep, and goats must be made instantaneously insensible to pain prior to slaughter.

If the plant is using one of Temple's designs correctly, humane slaughter is assured. "The cattle walk calmly down a gentle staircase until they find themselves supported by the chest and belly on a track Grandin designed. They see a diffused light shining above them and a moment later, a stunner renders them unconscious," reports Steve Warblow in *Cargill News*.

People for the Ethical Treatment of Animals (PETA) awarded Temple a Proggy award in 2004. This award goes to a person or group that has an innovative approach to the welfare of animals. "Years back the president of PETA was quoted in *The New Yorker* as crediting Temple with relieving more suffering (of animals) than anyone who'd ever lived," said Norm Ledgin, who wrote *Diagnosing Jefferson*.

From my interview with Mike Siemen, I learned Temple is an adviser and educator, but there's not much gray area. "It's either right or wrong," said Siemen.

If someone asks her a technical question, she may take half an hour to answer. She believes those who deal with factual details contribute far more to progress than people who engage in purely social exchanges such as "How's the weather?" and tend to be more constructive.

"I learned when talking on the phone with Temple about my manuscript *Diagnosing Jefferson* that if I wanted to win her help and support with the project, I'd better be more detailed in my writings about Jefferson," said Ledgin. She has no patience with beating around the bush. She likes facts, details, directness, and tends to get lost when others are vague or speak or write in abstract language.

Temple's insistence on facts and details has served her well in her capacity as a designer of humane handling of animals. Her focus on detail has also helped her develop standards for auditing meatpacking plants.

"Slaughter plants that have the best animal welfare standards are usually those that are audited by a major customer,"
Temple notes. In the United States, major customers such
as McDonald's, Wendy's, and Burger King audit large meat
plants. In the meat industry, Temple observed that measuring
and auditing greatly improved practices. "The percentage of
animals that vocalize (moo and squeal) should be measured
when observing cows and pigs," she wrote.[8]

The American Meat Industry guidelines were adapted from
those developed by Temple in the mid 1990s. Today there's a
committee, which both Mike Siemen and Temple are on, that
reviews the guidelines annually. The 2010 edition is 111 pages
long. Some years they're just tweaked, and sometimes major
changes are made.

Originally, biased audits—for example, moos counted by
a worker—were made with a clipboard. Today, checks are
also made with a remote video called "unbiased auditing."
The goal is to have them match within 2 percent of each other.
Reports are made every week. One group looks at the plants
and provides incentives for the plant that scores the highest.

For her animal welfare audit, Temple came up with five
key measurements that inspectors need to take to ensure cows
receive humane treatment at a meatpacking plant:

1. Percentage of animals stunned or killed correctly
   on the first attempt has to be at least 95 percent of
   animals.
2. Percentage of animals that remain unconscious after
   stunning must be 100 percent.
3. Animals that vocalize, squeal, bellow, or moo during handling and stunning should be no more than
   three cattle out of one hundred. Handling includes

walking through alleys and being held in the restraining device for stunning.

4. Animals that fall down, which terrifies them, should be no more than one out of one hundred.
5. Electric prod usage should be no more than 25 percent.

Consideration of employees is also important. Employees should not be constantly involved in killing, bleeding, or driving animals, so they need to be rotated. No one should constantly breathe the tainted air or be around so much death. "Complete automation of the actual killing procedure is good for employee well-being," Temple says. "Automation of killing is especially important in high-speed plants with rates of over 150 cattle per hour."[9]

Turnover in slaughter plant employees is understandably high, but it's "200 percent lower than it was in the 1980s," according to Temple. "It is essential not to overwork animal handlers or put them in a situation that is understaffed. Tired people will abuse animals. Internal unpublished data from large pig and poultry companies have shown that death and injuries doubled after crews had worked more than six hours."[10] Temple urges governments, non-government organizations (NGOs), animal activist groups, and livestock companies to support and educate fieldworkers and researchers. These people are essential to make real change, and then improvements take place.[11]

Ideally, management walks through the stunning area, constantly observing. "Well-designed facilities provide the tools that make humane handling possible. They are useless unless supervision and management go with them," said Temple.

Management attitude is the most important variable. The manager who enforces good animal handling is usually most effective if he is at the plant manager level.

"Grandin's battles in the slaughter industry have nearly all been waged with higher management, not with workers or floor managers, simply because they're office bound, their thinking determined more by the paper that surrounds them than by living animals and working plant," Verlyn Klinkenborg reported.[12]

For much of her career, Temple has been involved with pigs, probably the smartest animals among livestock. Winston Churchill said, "I like pigs. Dogs look up to us. Cats look down on us. Pigs treat us like equals."

Along with being highly intelligent, pigs are very social. They enjoy each other's company, but pigs also search for positive and close interaction with humans.

Mark Deesing, the only employee of Grandin Corporation, lives on a thirty-acre farm. He raises pigs, which he names. When I was there, he had Dick Cheney and George Bush.

"Mark loves his pigs," Conny Flörcke, Temple's graduate assistant, told me. When they're ready to slaughter, he puts both pigs in the stun box and gives them treats, so they'll be comfortable when it's time. He puts them in for a short time each day for several weeks before he actually kills them.

He stopped letting one boar watch while he slaughtered the other when he saw the watching pig shudder. "Now I put a blanket over the stun box so he can't see me as I butcher the other one," said Mark.

Pigs are obsessed with straw. "No one has found anything that can compete with straw for a pig's interest and attention," Temple noted.[13] "Each little flake of straw is different and fascinating, and the pigs are driven to explore and chew their straw until it's all gone. Both pigs and children with autism are obsessed with the things they like to manipulate."[14]

Temple recalled how as a child she endlessly ran grains of sand through her fingers, examining each one.

Sows produce a large litter for such a large animal. I remember seeing sows at the state fair nursing sixteen or more piglets.

A pig's pregnancy lasts three months, three weeks, and three days. When a sow lives in the wild, she leaves the group before farrowing and finds a suitable place to build a nest.

"At first when sows build a nest for their babies, it's a sloppy mess. Later it gets better," said Mark Deesing. "Maternal behavior starts with nest-building to provide the piglets with shelter, comfort, and to keep them warm, especially important for small piglets."[15] Sows have to learn to build nests.

Today sows are generally kept on cement. "A gestation stall is where a sow is kept confined during her entire pregnancy. The sow can lie down and stand up, but she cannot turn around," Temple explains.[16] Since pigs like to explore, these animals live in an environment that is extremely boring.

However, thanks to animal rights activists, things are changing. "Cargill Pork, based in Wichita, said . . . that its sow operations will use only group housing. . . . Group housing allows the sows to walk around and interact. Animal rights groups have convinced the public to demand that retailers and restaurant chains buy pork produced by farms that don't use gestation crates," the *Wichita Eagle* reported.[17]

The relationship between pigs and stockpersons is important in the plants, too. "The main aversive properties of humans for pigs include hitting, slapping, and kicking by the stockperson while rewarding acts include patting, stroking, and a hand of the stockperson resting on the back of the animal."[18]

"Human-animal interactions may markedly affect the behavior, productivity, and welfare of pigs. It's possible that the stockperson may be the most influential factor affecting pig-handling and animal welfare," Temple wrote.[19] Choosing stock people who relate well to animals and care about them is vital to plant operations.

Animals, processing industries, and plant employees have all benefitted from Temple's insights.

CHAPTER 16

MORE ABOUT ANIMAL WELFARE

My paternal grandmother, a chubby lady, always wore a print dress covered with an apron. Every morning and evening she walked to the henhouse to feed the chickens. She carried a pan with grain in it, which she generously distributed. Clucking and pecking chickens gathered around her.

During the day the chickens roamed freely, eating grasshoppers and various other bugs. They defecated wherever they wanted, so you had to be careful when stepping in the barnyard. If you weren't, you might be sorry.

At night Grandma shooed the hens into the chicken house and locked the door. A rooster always crowed early in the morning, signaling time to get up. The next day the routine repeated.

My immediate family also had chickens. When I was four, I watched my mother lay the head of a chicken on a tree stump and chop the head off with an ax. Blood spattered everywhere. The chicken flapped around, but Mama assured me it was dead. After all, the head was off. Then she dipped the chicken into boiling water and plucked off the feathers. The foul-smelling next step involved holding the chicken over the flame on a gas cooking stove to singe the remaining pin feathers.

When I was in third grade, I gathered eggs in the henhouse and sold them to buy my first bicycle. I used a long stick to pry a cantankerous hen off her egg, so I could grab it.

In the early 1960s, nearby neighbors farmed chickens commercially. I first glimpsed factory farming on their property. They had several huge chicken houses with caged chickens inside. The caged chickens had no freedom to wander. They were so crowded they stumbled over each other. They performed well in their job, laying eggs.

Temple Grandin doesn't have the fuzzy feelings for chickens that she has for cows, but she's concerned about the welfare of all animals. She said, "A factory farm is a huge outdoor facility or warehouse where the animals are treated like machines instead of thinking, feeling creatures."[1]

Factory farms have appeared because farming is too expensive for small farmers today. Daddy was concerned about giant corporate entities taking over the small farmers. "There's no way to compete," he said. "They're going to run the small farmer out of business." Small farms are rapidly disappearing. Most of our food animals are raised on factory farms. In the United States alone, there are ten billion food animals. Most of them are birds.

The chief aim of intensive egg producers is to make the chicken into a superefficient machine for laying more and more eggs in a given time. Intensive egg producers show a blatant disregard for the well-being of their chickens. Laying hens are spent in two years.

Temple wrote, "Laying hens probably have the worst welfare of any farm animal. Birds aren't covered by any federal humane slaughter laws. On most factory farms, hens are confined to a cage with other birds that is so cramped, each bird has less space than a sheet of paper."[2]

"Some of the farms just throw the hens when they are old ladies into dumpsters live. Others get rid of spent hens by sucking them up in a vacuum truck that is used to clean sewers," Temple reports.[3]

"Chickens are cheap, cages are expensive, so one crowds as many chickens into each cage as physically possible. Concentration of chickens requires huge amounts of antibiotics and other drugs to prevent wildfire spread of disease in overcrowded conditions," reports Bernard Rollin, an author writing about animal welfare.[4]

Drugs are used automatically in small quantities in the compounded chicken food to allow uninhibited growth, and in larger quantities to suppress disease when it appears. Synthetic hormones are used for fattening. As a result, food safety often suffers.

This raises a question: Do we know enough about these potent drugs to risk the hazard that some residue, however slight, will remain in the flesh or egg we then consume? We've heard a lot from medical authorities about only using antibiotics when necessary so they'll work when we really need them, but some agricultural authorities are encouraging ever wider use.

"We need to be selective about the drugs we use in animals and when we use them," said William Flynn of FDA's Center of Veterinary Medicine. "Antimicrobial resistance may not be completely preventable, but we need to do what we can to eliminate them."

* * *

For thousands of years, humans have used selective breeding to improve production of crops and livestock. This practice has rapidly increased recently. "The productivity of domestic livestock and poultry has almost tripled in the last hundred years through the use of both improved feeding methods and genetic selection," Temple Grandin and Mark Deesing report.[5] This benefits the owners, but the animals suffer.

"Breeders choose the most productive animals, the fastest-growing, the heaviest, the best egg layers and selectively breed just these animals. Bad things always happen when an animal is overselected for any single trait," Temple writes.[6]

"Whereas in traditional agriculture a milk cow could remain productive for ten and even fifteen years, today's milk cow lasts slightly longer than two lactations, a result of metabolic burnout and the quest for ever increasingly productive animals hastened by the hormone bovine estrogen (BST)," Bernard Rollin reports.[7] The cow lives in a confined animal feeding operation (CAFO) and leads a miserable life: crowded conditions, surrounded by manure, with nothing to do all day.

"In 1923 it took 16 weeks to produce a broiler chicken. In 1993 only 6.5 weeks were required," Temple and Mark Deesing reported.[8] "If you grew as fast as a chicken, you'd weigh 349 pounds at age two," they continue.[9]

Temple Grandin and Mark Deesing are both concerned that "the most serious animal welfare problems in the future may be caused by overselection for production traits such as rapid growth, leanness, and high milk yield."[10]

Another concern is the loss of genetic diversity. "Bill Muir, a genetics specialist at Purdue University, found that commercial lines of poultry have lost 90 percent of their genetic diversity compared to noncommercial poultry," Bernard Rollin reports.[11] This is alarming because genetically similar animals are more susceptible to disease. There are still farms where owners are concerned with the welfare of its animals. Good Shepherd Turkey Ranch, owned by Frank Reese, is dedicated to marketing Heritage Turkeys whose inherited traits are acceptable and diverse.

Reese defines a Heritage Turkey three ways. First, the turkey must be the result of naturally mating pairs of both grandparents and parents. Second, the Heritage Turkey must be able to reproduce for five to seven years for hens, and three to five years for toms. They also live outside. Although the turkeys are free to roam outside during the day, they're brought inside at night because of predators. Third, they reach a marketable weight in about twenty-eight weeks, comparable to growth rates of the twentieth century. The varieties raised by Good Shepherd include Standard Bronze, Bourbon Red Narragansett, Black Turkey, and White Holland.

Reese lives in Lindsborg, Kansas, though due to Kansas weather concerns, his turkeys are raised in several places. Turkeys are omnivores, so tall grass pastures provide a rich environment for the birds' food searches. Frank rotates the pastures to maintain healthy soil and grass. Outdoor and indoor nest boxes are provided for hens.

Fortunately, Reese is only one of a number of small breeders in the United States today. Small breeders are valuable for at least two reasons: First, "Keeping the classic breeds alive is the only way to preserve genetic diversity and to save animals that have valuable genetic traits breeders may want to breed back into commercial lines in the future," Temple writes, and second,[12] "The meat from some of the old breeds is tenderer and better quality than from animals bred for rapid growth and the chickens are hardier too."[13]

She concludes: "Many of the older breeds of poultry are being raised by local farmers and sold in farmer's markets or to gourmet restaurants. If a serious disease kills commercial broilers or layers, the entire world will be thanking the small producers."[14]

* * *

People concerned with the welfare of animals realize they need ways to motivate farmers and others to treat the animals better. One effective approach to persuade workers to treat animals better is by using economic incentives. "Reward animal handlers with extra pay for low levels of bruises, injuries, and deaths. In the U.S. and British poultry industries, broken wings were reduced from 5 percent to 1 percent by paying a bonus to chicken loaders when there were 1 percent or less broken wings, " *Improving Animal Welfare* reports.[15]

Financial incentives work around the world with all kinds of animals. "Parennas de Costa in Brazil reported that when supermarkets audited bruises and made deductions from transporters' pay, bruising was reduced from 20 percent to 1 percent of cattle," *Improving Animal Welfare* continues.[16] Carman Gallo in Chile also acknowledges that bruises were fewer when transporters received fines for injury to animals.

This financial incentive involves creative thinking. "One major chicken company has an interesting contract with the family farms that raise their chickens. The farms can't turn their chickens over to hired help. The reason for this is that the primary caretaker will get the extra money for taking good care of the chickens," one report states.[17] This profit benefits both the farmer and the chickens.

Another method to improve the conditions for animals involves consumer demands. "One huge positive force for improving animal welfare is that consumers are demanding that animals be treated better. Corporations both large and small can be motivated to improve practices when consumers demand it," reports Temple.[18]

Taking upper management on trips to see farms and slaughter plants can inspire improvement as well. "One executive became highly motivated to improve conditions after he saw an emaciated, sick old dairy cow going into his hamburger," Temple wrote.[19]

Handling practices need to be constantly measured to prevent them from increasingly deteriorating. Temple has given many seminars on low-stress handling and quiet movement of pigs and cattle. But sometimes when she returned to a farm a year later "many employees had reverted back to their old ways," she said.[20] As in many cases, the manager hadn't even noticed.

Sometimes she sends Mark Deesing to visit pork slaughterhouses. He visited one where they were slaughtering 12,000 animals a day. The numbers were daunting and the handling was terrible. It was difficult for Mark to keep his cool.

"Temple is always politically correct," he said. "She can close off emotional circuits in her brain. I can't. She promised to keep me out of nasty slaughterhouses as much as possible."[21]

Temple suggests using webcams to see what people are doing in plants and on farms when no one's looking. "Transparency has a powerful psychological effect because people and animals behave differently when they know someone is watching," she says.[22] Evidence supports this.

As the population of the world increases, more food will be needed to feed all the people. And this means faster and more production of poultry and meat will be needed. Brazil is already gearing up.

"At Granja Mantiqueira in Brazil eight million hens lay fifty-four million eggs a day. Conveyor belts whisk the eggs to a packaging facility. Demand for meat has tripled in the developing world in four decades, while egg consumption has increased *sevenfold*, driving a huge expansion of large-scale animal operations," *National Geographic* reports.[23] "Each month some 4.5 million chickens are killed, plucked, cut, trimmed and packaged at this plant near Sidrolândia, Brazil. Their parts will travel the globe."

Temple remains concerned about the welfare of animals, particularly as the need for more animals for food increases. In an excerpt from the Glass Wall Project, a video tour entitled *Turkey Farm and Processing Plant with Temple Grandin*, dated October 5, 2013, highlights the areas where she sees improvement.

Temple appears before us wearing a bouffant cap and gown. She explains that it's not practical to take people on a real tour of the farm and processing plant because of biosecurity issues. Biosecurity means "persistent threats to animal and public health from foreign animal diseases and emerging foodborne pathogens have elevated the importance of implementing sound biosecurity measures during livestock production," according to Temple.[24] "I had to be away from all birds for a week and then wear these clothes to keep the germs off," she says.

"These males are displaying to me as I walk through the barn," she says. "They are obviously comfortable. Someone has been walking through all the time." She explains that good management does this.

The turkeys move in small groups on a conveyor to ride in a truck. The conveyor has been a big improvement for the turkey industry. The birds are heavy. People get tired. Equipment doesn't.

The truck has fiberglass panels in it, which are removed in summer for ventilation and put back in for cold winter temperatures. The birds always have access to water. The truck is weighed with all the birds on it, then weighed again after all the birds are off.

Unloading is done in near darkness. Comfortable and quiet holding conditions reduce stress.

The birds are stunned unconscious in their cages before they are removed. They are bled and their heads taken off before they hit the scalder. Then most of the feathers are removed. Rubber fingers take off the pin feathers. In turkeys the innards are taken out by hand. A hose removes the feces.

Through her writing and speaking, Temple brings attention to the welfare of animals to corporations and, more importantly, the public. During the last thirty-five years, Temple has visited over five hundred farms and slaughter plants in thirty-five countries. In 2015 she spoke at approximately thirty animal welfare and animal behavior conferences in the United States. In 2016 she is traveling to England, Australia, and New Zealand for conferences.

"Temple landed at Colorado State University just as the stirrings of concern for animal welfare were beginning. They've been greatly accelerated by Temple," Bernard Rollin said. "She's brought a combination of thought and practicality, devotion to animals, and relationship to the industry unlike anybody else in the world."

PART IV

AUTISM AND ANIMALS

CHAPTER 17

DO ANIMALS THINK?

When I was a child, my great-aunt Myrtle, a petite woman with gray hair piled on her head, lived next door to us in a huge house in the country. On the occasions she hosted family dinners, my brother, my cousin, and I delighted in sliding down the long oak stairway railing in the middle of her home. Of course, we only did it when the adults weren't watching.

Aunt Myrtle lived alone because Uncle Bill had died of a heart attack only eighteen months after their marriage. Her first husband had also passed away shortly after they wed.

Living by herself terrified my great-aunt. Our family frequently took her home from church activities at night. Daddy walked her up to the door. Then Aunt Myrtle looked under every piece of furniture in the house while we waited in the car for what seemed like hours. At last she came out and waved us on.

Fortunately, she had a dog for protection and, more importantly, companionship. Her dogs were always black Scotties and always called "Babs." She insisted they could think and feel. Researchers have decided she was right.

Today many researchers admit that evidence is overwhelmingly in favor of those who contend that animals can think. Now the question is, "How and what do they think?"

Animals do not necessarily have language. Some scientists speculate that animals may think in images. Animals have sensory-based communication. They don't think with words as we do, but that doesn't mean they don't think. "Animals notice small sensory details that people often fail to notice. Since animals do not have verbal language, they are much more aware of tiny visual details in their environment people often fail to notice," Temple says.[1]

"Many or even most autistic people experience the world a lot [in] the way animals experience the world: as a swirling mass of tiny details," she says. "We're seeing, hearing, and feeling all the things no one else can."[2]

Some researchers believe human communication and animal communication are on the same spectrum. These researchers believe "animal language might turn out to be simpler than human language, the way a two-year-old's language is simpler than an adult's, but it's still language. The difference is quantitative, not qualitative," Temple notes.[3]

Some scientists don't want to admit that animals can have emotions. Temple disagrees. "The fact animals have emotions is well-documented," she says. "Their nervous systems are about the same as ours. They have the same chemicals in the brain."[4] Temple points out, "That's why your vet can prescribe the same antianxiety drug for your dog as he does for you." Not all vets know or at least admit this, but many do. "Animals and people have different brains, so they experience the world in different ways, but animals and people have an awful lot in common," she concludes.[5]

In graduate school at the University of Illinois, Temple dissected a human brain and a pig's brain and was shocked. "When I compared the lower-level structure like the amygdala to the same structures in the human brain, I couldn't see any difference at all. The pig brain and the human brain looked exactly alike."[6]

She had to look at the neocortex to see a difference. "The human neocortex is visibly bigger and more folded-up than the animal's, and anyone can see it. You don't need a microscope," she said.[7]

My husband Dave and I have lived with our cats, Chester and Dexter, long enough to see lots of evidence that they think and feel. Our certified vet-tech daughter, Lisa, gave them to me one year for Mother's Day. She thought we needed to fill our empty nest. When they arrived at our house, they were about nine weeks old.

Chester and Dexter are short-haired with white, gray, and black fur and heart-shaped faces like their mother. They both purr loudly and persistently. As kittens they sported extraordinarily long tails. "That means they're going to be big boys," Lisa told me. She was right.

I'd asked for two. I'd read in *Animals Make Us Human* by Temple that two cats keep each other company and two kittens from the same litter are best. Dexter is the dominant cat. I named him after my maternal grandfather. He came out of the carrier first and he always eats first. "Usually the dominant cat is the biggest and the oldest and almost always male," according to Temple. That definitely describes Dexter.

Dave named Chester, the sweeter one, after his dad. He follows Dave around and sits in Dave's lap. Chester runs to greet Dave when he comes home.

Chester and Dexter enjoy each other enormously. They wrestle, play, and stalk each other. They'll often curl up in the same chair to sleep. Frequently, one licks the other and his brother returns the favor.

Our cats sit on a chair by a spacious window so they can look out into several lawns behind us. They have a stand in front of the fireplace downstairs so they can sit on it, watch the fire, and be warm. Usually just one of them sits on it, but occasionally they sit side by side, with their long, raccoon-like tails hanging down.

Many times we are captivated by their antics. Dave often says, "Why do we need a television?" It takes little to entertain them. A string, a bag, or a box will do just fine. Chester finds his tail intriguing and will chase it round and round. Chester is fascinated by the cursor on the television and tries to attack it with his paw.

The garage enchants Dexter and he spends many happy times exploring it. Dexter dotes on kitty treats. He quickly found them when I hid them in a drawer in the kitchen. I felt foolish when hiding them in a drawer in the bedroom, but I was almost certain he wouldn't find them there. I was wrong. Dexter acts like he can tell time and frequently comes and sits in front of me when it's time to eat.

The "boys" sniff anything new brought into the house or even anything moved just a little. We understand the saying, "Curiosity killed the cat."

We are also convinced pets need human friendship. Dexter and Chester are usually in the same room with us, or nearby. Chester especially seems to need to be close to us. They enjoy each other's company, but apparently they crave ours, too.

Temple said, "People constantly underestimate domestic animals' need for companionship. Most experts believe that the reason these animals became domesticated was that they were highly social. All domestic animals need companionship."[8]

Obviously, we are very connected to the boys. They've given us companionship, entertainment, and affection. They're young now, but eventually one of them will pass on. Inevitably, we will grieve.

There are support groups for people who've lost pets. When the time comes that we lose one of our boys, we'll probably join one.

I remember how I felt when Lisa and I took Smokey, our first cat, to the vet for the last time. He was gasping for air, but he seemed to be saying, "Thank you for a good life." Lisa and I both had tears rolling down our faces when we left him. Magic, our second cat, mourned Smokey's loss also. Magic never recovered and died shortly afterward.

Pets feel sad when their owners die, too. *Reader's Digest* gives an example: "In Montagnana, Italy, after Ilzzelli Renzo died, his cat placed items on his grave for months. Renzo had adopted the cat from a shelter when he was three months old and the two became inseparable. After Renzo passed away, the kitty followed the coffin to the cemetery. Now the cat guards the grave."

Sadness is not the only emotion that animals show. Another emotion animals demonstrate is compassion. Just like people, some animals are undoubtedly more empathetic than others, but a few have remarkable empathy.

Charlie, a blind horse, and Jack, a goat, met at Wild Heart Ranch near Claremore, Oklahoma, owned by Annette Tucker. When Charlie lost his sight, Annette put him in a pen so he wouldn't wander off and get lost. Then she telephoned the veterinarian to put him down. The vet was busy and took a few days to arrive. Jack started leading Charlie around.

Annette called the vet and said, "We have a seeing-eye goat." Jack led Charlie for sixteen years, even though Jack was a lazy goat and Charlie was an active horse. "Some animals have self-appointed jobs," said Annette.

Relationships make us healthier. Friendships help us survive. Tighter social bonds lower stress levels. Many people find deep friendship with animals.

Most pet owners say companionship, love, company, and affection are the main benefits to owning a pet. If you live with animals, you know that the animals have many of the same attributes.

Great-Aunt Myrtle was not alone.

CHAPTER 18

RABBITS AND AUTISM

Seven-year-old Chris, who has autism, entered the room hesitantly. He appeared lost in his own world. Joyce Gedraitis, who has a bunny club, happened to be at the respite care center that night when his mother dropped him off. The rabbit fascinated Chris. He watched it quietly. Joyce read a book about bunnies to the group. Slowly, Chris reached out and touched the rabbit. He read the story about the bunny aloud to the group. As he interacted with the bunny, his attitude changed. When his mom came to pick up Chris, she was amazed at the change in him.

There is nothing quite like a loving, trusting creature up against you. A rabbit seems to know when somebody needs him. Just the simple pleasure of having a bunny sit quietly in your lap is intensely soothing. A bunny's unconditional acceptance makes the child—whether special needs or neurotypical—feel included and loved.

A rabbit is safe and nonthreatening. Children who are afraid of dogs or horses often benefit from connecting with a rabbit. Interaction with a rabbit teaches empathy for living things, which children with autism lack. They can learn how to read body language. Animals do not mask feelings the way humans do, making it easy to read them. They give the child with autism spectrum disorders (ASD) the opportunity to look outside himself and at the surrounding environment.

Studies have shown that interaction with animals sparks social interaction and laughter. Studies have also shown that interaction with rabbits breaks down barriers. Children with ASD are more relaxed and willing to talk during or after animal visits.

Therapy animals are a relatively new idea, and this is especially true with rabbits. Some kinds of rabbits are well-suited for therapy. "American Sable, Angora, and mini-Rex are docile and love human attention. Female Dutch rabbits are excellent mothers and this nurturing can extend to humans. American Chinchilla and Flemish Giant help people open up and interact with the world around them," says Diana David in *Rabbit Examiner*.

There are two types of placement for therapy rabbits. The first is when a team brings a rabbit to a facility such as a school, nursing home, or community group for hands-on learning and interaction. TenderLovingEars.webs.com also places a rabbit with an individual or family on a permanent basis.

Rabbits have a long lifespan, more than ten years, and many specific requirements. If your family wants a rabbit, research rabbit care through books and websites. Rabbits need a bunny-savvy veterinarian. For behavioral and health reasons, they should be spayed or neutered.

Our daughter Michelle loved the touch of soft things, especially fur. After I bought her a pink fur coat when she was in first grade, she slept with it for a week. We weren't surprised when she asked for a pet bunny. We bought Midnight, a black d white rabbit from Michelle's friend who was raising show rabbits for 4-H. We got a cage, rabbit pellets, and a water bottle, but had little understanding of the rabbit's needs.

"Pet rabbits need to be let out regularly to hop about, explore, and feel the ground under their feet, just as a wild rabbit does when it comes out of its burrow to forage for food. And they need company, because it is natural for rabbits to live in groups. A rabbit kept on its own will be lonely unless it gets a lot of human companionship," writes Helen Piers in *Taking Care of Your Rabbit*.[1]

"A pet rabbit's food is brought to it, but it will get bored and even bad-tempered unless it is let out of its hutch often to run about and explore," she continues.[2] Midnight got grumpy because we did not let him out often enough. We also didn't give him enough companionship, human or rabbit. According to experts, two sister rabbits from the same litter are best.

Other pet rabbit care information:

1. A rabbit's front teeth grow up to one-half inch a month. "Find a small tree branch for your rabbit to gnaw on. Gnawing keeps the teeth healthy. A branch from an untreated fruit tree is best," says Mark Evans in *A Practical Guide to Caring for Your Rabbit*.[3]
2. "Rabbits eat their own droppings so that they pass through their body a second time. This is to make sure they get all the good they can from their food," writes Judith Heneghan in *Love Your Rabbit (Your Perfect Pet)*.[4]
3. A bunny can easily be litter box trained. Place the rabbit in a litter box, such as one used for cats, every few minutes. It won't be long before the rabbit learns to go to the box on its own. Don't expect a cat

and a rabbit to share the same litter box. Give each a litter box of its own. Clay, straw, wood chips, and garden dirt can all be used for litter. Experiment to see which your rabbit prefers.

4. Your rabbit should always have fresh hay and water available. Give him rabbit pellets twice a day. Spread out one-eighth to one-quarter cup for each five pounds of body weight.

5. Variety is important. Feed your bunny fresh green vegetables such as collard greens, arugula, and endive. Note: pesticides shouldn't be on dandelion greens or anything given to a rabbit to eat.

6. Rabbits enjoy treats. Treats should be given occasionally and in moderation. Fresh carrots are a treat and so are apples, but no apple seeds.

7. Rabbits don't overeat. If food that will spoil is left over, just throw it away and give less next time.

8. Rabbits need a warm, clean shelter either indoors or outdoors for sleeping and hiding. A rabbit's cage should be thoroughly scrubbed every two weeks.

9. Short-haired rabbits need to be brushed twice a week. Long-haired rabbits shed more hair and need to be brushed daily.

10. "A rabbit should spend most of the day outside its cage. When your rabbit is in its cage, give it some toys to play with. Playing with toys will keep it from getting bored," write Kelley MacAulay and Bobbie Kalman in *Rabbits*.[5]

11. Change the toys often. Put empty cardboard toilet paper rolls and empty cardboard paper towel rolls in the cage to chew on. Sometimes add a treat in the

middle of the empty roll. Give your pet something new to investigate every week: logs to hop on, cardboard boxes to hide in, or balls to nudge.

In the wild, rabbits are hunted by predators. Don't be surprised when a domestic bunny is afraid. Let your rabbit get used to your smell before picking it up. "Practice picking up your rabbit while kneeling on the ground until you are confident. Then if you drop him, he won't get hurt," says one rabbit expert.

"It is important to handle your rabbit for a short time every day if possible. Talk to him and call him by name. He will get to know his name and the sound of your voice."[6] Don't overtire your rabbit by handling it too long.

Joyce Gedraitis, who has owned rabbits for more than twenty years, started a bunny club called TNT in Wichita, Kansas. TNT stands for Training, Nurturing, Therapy. She hoped to inspire rabbit owners to train their pets as therapy animals. She also wanted bunny owners to have a chance to share with each other the joys and trials of owning a rabbit.

Meetings were a time for bunnies to get together and enjoy the company of other furry friends. She planned events like a Birthday Bash, where members taught guests about bunnies. There were bunnies for petting and an art project for children.

Joyce got her first rabbit when her daughter was fifteen. Now her husband, John, and daughter, Joan, and Joyce all have rabbits they have shared with other people in the community. Joan took her rabbit, Elizabeth, to a variety of groups in Kansas City. One of the places she visited was for visually impaired students. The soft fur of the rabbit, its long delicate ears, and its twitchy nose were all a rich palette of learning for visually impaired children.

John's bunny, Rosebud, played Easter bunny for six years at the Arc of Sedgwick County Kansas's annual Easter egg hunt. The Arc serves persons with special needs. Rosebud was very social. "She would lie down and spread out as far as she could to make room for lots of little hands," said John.

Once a week for three years, Joyce visited Brendan Duncan, a severely disabled man. She took a rabbit, Cinnamon, with her, sharing her love for bunnies with a person in the community who needed a little unconditional love. Brendan loved the rabbit. It gave him something to look forward to and something to talk about. "It makes him think about other things besides the normal whatever's going on around here. The more he thinks the better," said Georgia Duncan, Brendan's mom. Brendan's conversational speech improved. "He anticipates, he knows what's coming next, he carries on more of a conversation," said Joyce.

Bunnies also visit nursing homes with pet owners. "The clients would visit with the rabbit when they wouldn't interact with other people," said Joyce.

The House Rabbit Society keeps a list of basic bunny facts that Bunny TNT likes to share:

1. Rabbits can purr when contented.
2. Like cats and dogs, rabbits need to be spayed or neutered to improve health and behavior.
3. Most rabbits do not like to be held. They prefer to sit beside you.
4. Rabbits need to have things of their own to chew on (or they will nibble on your stuff).
5. Rabbits need to be protected from predators, poison, temperature extremes, electrical cords, and rough handling.

Bunny TNT recognizes that a child with autism may benefit from a bunny in many ways. Treatment is not as scary as pills or needles, but care can be time-consuming. It also can be a cuddly and effective form of treatment for autism that benefits the whole family.

CHAPTER 19

CATS AND DOGS AND AUTISM

People with autism face communication difficulties every day. Much has been written about the benefits of dogs and horses for people with autism. Cat therapy is only beginning to be explored.

Cats are smaller than dogs and not as noisy. Many youngsters with Asperger's have sensitive hearing and don't like a lot of noise. Samuel, who is fourteen and has Asperger's, described his experience in *Service Cats for Autism*, which was published online. Samuel said, "I have a service cat named Hub and he has saved my life. Not every cat can be a service cat. They have to have the right personality for it. I have trained two (cats), so I know how to train them." He offered to train cats for others.

People with Asperger's need some living being to connect with who understands and serves as a mentor on communication. Cats are patient and use body language that the person must learn to translate into words and ideas, a struggle for those with autism. A cat can alert its owner to danger by sitting on his chest to get attention or using its claws to warn him.

George is a four-year-old autistic child. George and Pushkin the cat are friends. Inside they ignore each other, but when they're outside, Pushkin guards George. Pushkin shows George where the limits are. Pushkin claws George's mother or Sophie, George's sister, but never George. He apparently realizes George is different.

Pushkin could easily outrun George, but for whatever reason, he trusts George. When a spider appears, it's a race. Whoever gets to the spider first, eats it.[1]

According to Temple Grandin, "The sensitive period for socialization is the second week of a kitten's life to the seventh week, and the more people who handle the kitten during this time the better."[2] This recommendation from Temple comes as a suggestion for obtaining a cat with a friendly, bold temperament.

Temple Grandin is right. We do need "all kinds of minds." Cat therapy is a definite possibility for persons with autism.

Dogs, social and eager to please, can be very helpful to a person with autism. Temple said, "Dogs are so tuned in to people that they are the only animals that can follow a person's gaze or pointing finger to find out where a piece of food is hidden."[3]

A dog can do wonders for a child's social skills. A dog accepts a child just the way he is, and sometimes a child with autism may love his dog in ways he cannot love a person. Hopefully this transfers to others.

I met Clint at Camp SSTAR, an Asperger's day camp at Heartspring, where I volunteered when he was eight. Clint has greatly benefited from having Micah, a service dog. She's been a marvelous friend to him, giving him companionship and comfort. She wears a special vest that says "ask to pet," so children and adults inquire if they can pet her. This encourages social interaction, which is difficult for Clint.

There are three younger children in this family, to whom Micah relates well. She provides stress relief and a therapeutic presence for the whole family. In public, though, she knows her primary responsibility is Clint.

Micah aids in a number of ways. Clint's mother, Sherry, said, "Clint doesn't have as many meltdowns as he did before Micah came. He's calmer and more focused."

Besides autism, Clint has a seizure disorder, which his dog also helps with, alerting Clint that a seizure is coming as much as an hour before it happens. Micah runs to Sherry and then to Clint. If he has a seizure, Micah makes sure he stays away from dangerous places, such as the swimming pool or stairway. After a seizure, with the command of "brace," Micah stands straight and still so Clint can pull himself up.

"The seizure alert dogs use advanced perceptual abilities to solve a problem no dog was born knowing how to solve," Temple says. "Seizure alert dogs are dogs who can predict a seizure before it starts. There's still controversy over whether you can train a dog to predict seizures and so far people haven't had a lot of luck trying. But there are a number of dogs who have figured it out on their own. These dogs were trained as seizure-response dogs, meaning they can help a person once a seizure has begun.

"But some of these dogs have gone from responding to seizures to perceiving signs of a seizure ahead of time. No one knows how they do this, because the signs are invisible to people. No human being can look at someone who's about to have a seizure and see (or hear, smell, or feel) what's coming."[4] Perhaps dogs can detect a smell or smells indicating a seizure is coming on.

Micah was trained by Canine Assistance Rehabilitation Services (CARES), a nonprofit organization in Concordia,

Kansas. CARES is one of only five percent of canine assistance schools that accepts applications from children and adults with multiple disabilities. Founded in 1994 by Sarah Holbert, CARES has placed dogs across thirty-seven states and in several foreign countries including Peru, Puerto Rica, Belgium, and Latvia.

CARES trains dogs for people who need help with hearing assistance, juvenile diabetes, and autism. They don't train dogs to lead the sight impaired.

CARES gets its service dogs in several ways: retired show dogs, specifically bred puppies, and family pets. After initial testing such as temperament testing and health checks, a potential service dog is accepted into the program. Foster homes raise the puppy or dog from nine to eighteen months. In the home, they learn basic obedience and are socialized to public and private life. The dog accompanies his foster parent everywhere—to the grocery store, mall, work, restaurants, school, and church. He is expected to behave.

A variety of individuals and families volunteer to be foster parents. There are also specialized programs such as Tipton Academy, Ellsworth Correctional Facility, and El Dorado Correctional Facility that function as foster homes for these dogs. Puppy raisers are required to fill out a monthly progress report. CARES staff tracks the dog's progress.

After the basic socialization, assistance dogs are reevaluated for temperament and physical soundness. In the final phase of training, the dog learns to meet specific needs of his potential partner. Then the CARES staff finds the right dog to match the person's personality, lifestyle, and need.

The dog and his partner train together for ten days. Then there is a graduation ceremony. For the first six months, the client has temporary ownership, although CARES can take the dog back any time if it receives at least two reports of abuse.

"The dog is worth his weight in gold," said Megan Llewellyn, assistant canine director for the program.

Jim Sinclair, an adult with autism and founder of Autism Network International, was the pioneer who expanded the use of service dogs or "social signal dogs" into autism spectrum disabilities, beyond the conventional association with assisting the blind.

Jim writes: "I hoped a dog could help make it safer for me to get around. At that time it was not uncommon for me to walk off curbs into the street, or walk past my house without realizing it and find several blocks later that I didn't know where I was, or fail to hear a bicycle coming up behind me until it almost ran into me."

Jim was unable to find a place willing to train a dog for an autistic person, so he trained one himself. Isosceles, the fourth dog he coached, has been the best service dog that Jim has ever had. He performs routine guiding and signaling tasks that improve Jim's orientation and safety in the community. He also has social responsiveness.

"Isosceles has enabled me to recognize acquaintances when I encounter them, which has made it easier for acquaintances to turn into friends. He has helped to initiate some social contacts by noticing when someone was interested in meeting us. I am more oriented to my social environment as well as my physical environment," Jim said.

Isosceles has also helped Jim as he worked in schools. "I have worked with young, active, impulsive, unpredictable children who are autistic or have other developmental disabilities. And Isosceles has been right there with me: guiding me through noisy crowded hallways, signaling the right classrooms so I don't miss them, picking my clients out of the crowds until I learn to recognize them by myself, and patiently and cheerfully enduring the attentions of dozens of children.[5]

"Isosceles has developed the rare ability to pay attention to other people in the social environment, *without* losing his focus on me. It is important to me that Isosceles be aware of people and cues in the social environment, so that he can signal me in turn. I can allow people in my social world to pet Isosceles, and I can allow Isosceles to respond to them, because I know that if I make even the slightest movement, Isosceles will return his full attention to me to see if I need him. This is an extraordinary ability."[6]

The first agency that placed skilled autism service dogs, 4Pawsforability, has a satisfied parent who says this:

"I had to share what is happening to us. To bring the rest of you up to speed, we have an eight-year-old high-functioning son. We got our dog last March. Our son had *never, never* slept in his own bed. His 'security item' or 'transitional object' has always been Dad or me. So success number one: for the last two months he has been sleeping in his own bed with Popeye. No crying, no muss, no fuss."

Another comment from 4Paws:

"When a child with autism disappears, his life is in danger and an adult looking for him may begin a search in the wrong direction; a 4Paws Autism Assistance dog trained in search and rescue never takes the wrong path and quickly leads the adult to the missing child." (In an online survey conducted by the National Autism Association, an incredible 92 percent of respondents said their child was at risk of wandering. Wandering can occur anywhere, anytime. 4Paws is unique in training dogs to track a child who has disappeared.)

Terri Wible and her husband, Ken, have two adopted children, six months apart. Both are on the autism spectrum.

She says, "Adrianna has the first autism service dog we are aware of in the Kansas City area. We have had an autism service dog in our home since November of 2011. Adi has decreased from three to four violent meltdowns a day to two to three minor ones a month. She knows when she gets anxious or overwhelmed that her service dog Grady is there to help. Grady now recognizes when she is getting overstimulated. He focuses on her and disrupts the meltdown before it starts. Our family has begun to really enjoy public outings. Adrianna will now talk to people when they ask her about her working dog."

In thinking about getting an assistance dog, Temple Grandin said the first question to ask is "Does the child like dogs?" "There are three kinds of reactions the child can have: The first is an almost magical connection with dogs. The child and the dog are best buddies. They love being together. The second type of reaction is a child who may be initially hesitant, but learns to really like dogs. The third type of reaction is avoidance or fear."[7]

Temple also cautions: "Unlike other autism interventions that can be easily started and stopped, embarking on a journey to find an appropriate service dog for a child is a long-term commitment on the part of the entire family. A service dog is much more than a well-trained pet. . . . Parents must be willing and able to make the time, financial . . . and emotional commitment of having a service dog. This is a family affair with everyone in the family involved."[8]

Nevertheless, the right service dog in the right family may indeed be worth his weight in gold. When it comes to persons with autism, the fact that dogs know just what their partners need is nothing less than magical.

CHAPTER 20

HORSES AND AUTISM

As an adolescent, Temple loved horse riding. She, along with many other teenagers, escaped from the world of school problems into horseback riding. "Horses are super-sensitive to their riders and are constantly responding to the riders' needs without being asked," she wrote.[1]

People and horses should be together. "Even more so people on the autism spectrum and horses should be together. Both people and horses benefit from this special relationship," writes Alicia Kershaw, founder and director of Gallop New York City.

Research into animal-assisted therapy is fairly new. There's general consensus that therapy animals can be a highly beneficial addition to the treatment program for children with autism or Asperger's. Equine-assisted therapy seems to have the best results.

Many benefits come from horseback riding. The gentle rhythmic movement helps the rider improve balance, muscle control, and coordination. The rider brushes, hugs, and pats the horse. Tactile senses are stimulated. The horse's skin is fuzzy, the mane and tail are rough, and the nose is soft.

Riders are taught how to care for a horse as well as ride them. Grooming such as brushing, bathing, and currying develops the relationship. This helps the student see the world from a different perspective. Since persons with autism have walls that can be hard to penetrate, this is a valuable lesson.

Children often make eye contact with the horse first and then other people. Many autistic children have said their first words on horseback. Once again, the child talks to the horse first and then to other people.

"Language develops because repetitive rocking motion requires the person to continually find and refind his balance, which stimulates areas where learning receptors are located," said Temple.[2]

"Even people with severe autism can do well with riding. Horses calm riders with autism, allowing them to focus, think, and accept training. Desire to ride also allows encouraging positive behaviors and gently discouraging negative behaviors," said Alice Kershaw.

Kershaw grew up on a farm in upper New York State where she spent a lot of time with horses. As an adult she married, had three children, and obtained a law degree. At forty-five, she was a director at Merrill Lynch when she took a sabbatical to go with her husband, Peter, to Hong Kong. While overseas, she volunteered for a therapeutic riding group for special needs kids. It changed her life. When she came back to the United States, she started a therapeutic riding group in New York City.

"We teach riding in a careful and supportive way," said Kershaw. "A trained volunteer leads each rider's mount, and two volunteers walk either side of the horse to ensure the rider's safety. A certified instructor leads all classes. He or she has specialized training in Therapeutic Horsemanship."[3]

"We set individual goals for each rider and patiently work on skills such as speech, socialization, and fitness. And, yes, one of our goals is 'just pure fun,'" she adds.[4]

It is fun. While riding, children toss colorful balls into baskets. Singing a song while riding, they touch eyes, ears, nose, mouth, and chin. Riding helps children become excited and motivated to talk. They communicate with each other and with the animal.

And just as a child benefits from the horse, the horse tries to help the child. "The sociability of horses gives them a desire to please their human owners," says Temple. "When a horse has a good relationship with his rider, he has a built-in natural desire to cooperate and follow his rider's lead."[5]

"Real riding is a lot like ballroom dancing or maybe figure skating in pairs. It's a relationship," said Temple. "A good rider and his horse are a team. It's not a one-way relationship."

Like all animals, horses also have needs. "Horses are herd animals with strong social needs. Horses need companions," said Temple.[6] "Horses stand alongside each other, with each horse's head next to the other horse's butt, flicking flies from each other's faces. . . . When horses groom each other, their heart rates go down."[7]

Horses need other horses, but they also need human company. "People constantly underestimate domestic animals' need for companionship. Why did wild horses decide it was okay to have people sitting in a saddle on their backs holding a pair of reins?" Temple asked.[8]

Horses and people decided centuries ago that they need each other. There are cautions, though. "A horse is all about flight, and fear is the dominant emotion. Horses are much more flighty than other herd animals such as cows, sheep, or goats," said Temple.[9]

If horse riding is part of your life or your child's life, it's wise to know the signs of fear. "A fearful horse switches his tail. As he becomes more scared, the tail moves faster. Other signs are a high head, sweating when there is little physical exertion, and quivering skin. A really frightened horse gets bugged-out eyes and the whites show," reports Temple.[10]

"Horses sometimes startle when they see the same object from a different angle. The object looks different and therefore becomes a new, scary thing," reports Temple.[11] She goes on to say she does the same thing. She compares her way of seeing things and high level of anxiety with that of a horse.

One detriment to therapy with horses is that "horseback riding is dangerous even with a well-trained horse. One study of horseback riding injuries in England found that riding horses was twenty times more dangerous than riding motorcycles," reports Temple.[12] A helmet, help mounting the horse, three volunteers, and a trained instructor with the rider at all times are intended to minimize accidents in horse therapy.

Another detriment is the cost. Horse therapy is expensive. Parents of children with autism can find themselves paying over $5,000 annually for therapy lessons with horses. Although some organizations will help pay for lessons, children with autism already have many expenses, and this added expense can be prohibitive.

Owning a horse is costly, too. Buying a horse is just the beginning. Vet bills, hay, feed in the winter, and pasture in the summer all cost money. So does boarding the horse. Kathy Nunemaker, MA, CCC, has worked as a speech therapist since 1976 and has been involved in horse therapy since the 1990s. She bought Junta, an eighteen-year-old former polo horse, in 2007. Now Junta is a therapy horse.

Kathy and Junta took lessons where Junta learned how to trot, turn in a circle, and move her body in a more comfortable way. Kathy learned how to exercise Junta and how to communicate with her by the way she moved her body and hands. She learned the basics of horse care: how to retrieve a horse from the pasture, groom a horse, and saddle it. She also learned how to take care of a wound, take care of a sick horse, and play with a horse. They both enjoyed the lessons.

Kathy and I visited Junta at her barn in the mountains near Loveland one summer. Kathy has been acquainted with horses for a long time. She and Lois Hickman, MS, OTR, have done numerous camps and workshops for autistics. They were two of the first advocates of horse therapy.

When we visited Junta, Kathy groomed Junta, fed her treats, took the mud out of her hooves, and checked the hoof that had had a nail in it. Kathy said, "It's a marvelous place to board a horse. The boarders are like a family." She also told me that Junta is the leader of the pack at the place where she boards. "The other horses follow her lead."

Junta volunteers to be a therapy horse whenever she gets a chance. Kathy talks to Junta about the person she will be working with. "I told her about the teenager. I said, 'Be honest with him. Do only what he asks you to do.'" Junta walked stoically beside Kathy, listening to what she was saying. Junta seemed to know the importance of her job.

Kathy has personal experience with the benefits of horse therapy. She writes: "My own daughter, Eryn, was my first teacher on this journey. She started riding at Colorado Therapeutic Riding Center (CTRC) when she was three and a half years old, after it was discovered that she had a sensory integrating disorder that made her hypersensitive to touch and hard for her to sit still.

"Initially she wasn't very enthusiastic about the riding. We talked with her occupational therapist, Tamera, about her tactile defensiveness and how it affects many other areas of her life; how she had difficulty with light touch and how she would react often suddenly and aggressively to other children brushing past her. Tamera decided to include Eryn in the care of a horse. She talked to Eryn about how horses need brushing daily and always before and after riding. She also explained that you never surprise a horse by coming up from behind or you might get kicked. Eryn had found another being whose responses and needs were like her own, and her interest was definitely established.

"We started noticing subtle changes in her. She would not get upset as easily or as often. When she did get upset, she could come down faster. In the next year or two, I started to notice the subtleties of language that Eryn had experienced difficulty with were improving. However, because of tight schedules, Eryn's father and I decided to stop the riding when Eryn was in first grade. Within a few weeks, we noticed regression in her behavior and communication and we were convinced of the powerful therapeutic value of riding for our daughter. We enrolled her in the next session and she has been riding ever since.

"Seeing the improvement with Eryn, I began to suspect that the horses, with their power, grace and gentleness might offer a special therapeutic element to others with special needs."[13]

Ten-year-old Roger had difficulty with auditory processing, but was very bright and needed intellectual challenges. He had never ridden a horse before. Riding motivated him, encouraging him to listen to the instructor for directions and to his volunteer for additional cues when he needed them. He could stay focused on the task only if just one volunteer talked to him.

Having two volunteers talking, even if they took turns, was too confusing. Once he learned some basic skills, the therapist was able to give him more complex directions. His teacher was pleased when he could follow directions in the classroom.[14]

This is a typical lesson for ten-year-olds receiving horse therapy:

1. Meet the children at the front door. Do brushing proprioception, and then following directions.
2. They find their helmets and go out to the mounting area.
3. They might practice posting on the vaulting barrel or on a chair.
4. After mounting, they do exercises on the horse, while moving and sometimes sitting backwards on the horse.
5. Next they might do some start/stop with the music and/or practice a new riding skill, i.e. posting.
6. The next activity might be to follow complex auditory directions with the obstacles in the area.
7. Next they might play a game that requires good breath support and listening skills (i.e. wiggly worm, etc.) or review new terms learned or remember what activities they did during the session.

Not all horses are suitable for therapy. Horses need to have a solid work ethic, enjoy people, and be healthy and sound. A great therapy horse is sound at the walk, trot, and canter with three rhythmic and balanced gaits. Other qualities required include experience, good vision, trained, quiet, and at least six years of age. Riders vary in needs, so horses must also be varied to meet those needs.[15]

Horses bring different sizes, colors, and talents to the stable. Just like people, horses come from a wide variety of backgrounds, making for a diverse mix of body types, personalities, and skills. Puddin', a Palomino pony at CRTC, is popular with the riders, staff, and volunteers. His best qualities are wisdom and versatility. He adapts well to the needs of different riders.

Caesar's short legs keep him close to the ground, but his strength of character, good sense, and dependability more than make up for a lack of height and speed. Obe, a bay, has cross-country and hunter/jumper experience. He and Harry, a chestnut thoroughbred, fly over fences. The athletic abilities of these and others enhance the riding experience of all the students and truly challenge the more independent riders.

These equine therapists have tangible and intangible gifts to give. Each member of the herd is a unique treasure with his own tale to tell. The horses' willingness and unlimited hearts have captured the hearts of those who know them.

Good horsemen are talented observers of horse behavior and respond consistently to the horse's subtle cues. Learning the difference between individual horses and how they react to different situations is the key.

"As a rider learns that he can have control of a horse, he begins to learn he can take control of himself as well. Trust, impulse control, self-confidence, relationship building and natural consequences are all among the lessons learned. Opportunity to give verbal commands to the horse has allowed many of our riders to improve their verbal skills. They gain confidence to get on a horse, or the ability to navigate around a barrel, or trot once around the ring. Each week anywhere from 170 to over 200 riders achieve their goals with the aid of committed volunteers, instructors, and exceptional therapy horses," said Jane Harder of Reins of Hope in Hutchinson, Kansas.

Therapeutic riding is offered in a group setting of three to five riders once a week for one hour and one rider for thirty minutes. Instructors work diligently to create lesson plans that challenge each student and provide one-on-one attention and instruction. Therapeutic riding truly creates a bond among horse, rider, instructor, and volunteers.

I observed Jane's class one hot summer morning. The horse barn was remarkably cool and free of flies. A multitude of fans whirled on the ceiling. Two huge, open windows on opposite sides of the barn allowed the air to flow freely between them. The rider only mounted the horse with supervision. To mount, each child strapped on a helmet, sometimes with help, and climbed the stairs. Five horses, each with a volunteer on either side, followed one another tranquilly.

Even horses who know nothing about being a therapy horse show remarkable traits. Becky Tanner, a reporter for the *Wichita Eagle*, interviewed Debbie Yeager after her horse protected the other animals on her farm.

Jazz, a nine-year-old paint mare, saved animals in a bad storm. When the sky turned green, Jazz herded ducks, pigs, goats, cows, and horses into a small pen in the barn. Soon baseball-sized hail pelted down. Trees doubled over. Shingles flew off the house. After the storm, Jazz let the animals out of the pen. One by one, they marched out.

Tanner also interviewed Temple Grandin. Temple said it would be normal behavior for the horse to feel protective. "It happens quite commonly for an animal to protect another animal or person. Animals will protect one another, particularly where they sense weather change," said Temple. "I've seen cattle jump gates twelve hours before the big storm hits. It's the barometric pressure. They sense a bad storm coming."

Therapy horses protect their riders, and provide them with comfort. They teach their riders how to interact with animals and other people, and help them grow. As one rider says, "They're better than any human friend."

PART V

TEMPLE NOW

CHAPTER 21

HBO MOVIE

"I was hugging everybody that night," said Temple, speaking about the night the HBO movie, *Temple Grandin*, won seven Emmys.[1] She wore her usual Western wear, but she had on a Ralph Lauren cowboy shirt her sister had given her. The 2010 Emmys happened to be August 29, 2010—Temple's sixty-third birthday. What a wonderful way to celebrate a birthday!

Mark Deesing, Temple's only employee, co-author, and friend, said, "Temple told me about the HBO movie ten years ago, but didn't say anything again until eight years later. Then she called me and said, 'Pack your bags, you're going to Austin.' She'd already been through two rewrites and lots of consultations."

The movie tells Temple's story. Temple shrank from touch as a baby and through young adulthood. She developed from a child disconnected from the world, fixated on dribbling sand through her fingers and smearing her feces on the wall, to a woman world-renowned in two fields, autism and animal handling. Mick Jackson, director of the movie, said, "You couldn't write this as fiction. No one would believe it."

The movie begins with Temple's arrival in Arizona following her high school graduation. She is fascinated by a device that holds cows still. One day she crawls into it to stop a panic attack. Since Temple has sensory integration dysfunction, she dislikes physical affection from people. However, she finds the squeeze machine calming and she can control it. Temple takes it to college with her, but must prove it was only for calming herself. She graduates from Franklin Pierce College second in a class of four hundred. Then the movie shows her early struggles in her chosen career. In the 1970s she is the only woman in a man's world of cattle handling, rodeos, and ranching. Among her early projects, she rebuilds a dip vat and alters a slaughterhouse for cows to make it more humane. The movie finishes as she and her mother attend the 1981 Autism Society of America convention. Temple spontaneously explains much about autism to an eager audience.

Emily Gerson Saines, the executive producer of the movie, has a son diagnosed with autism. Her mother and grandmother gave Emily *Thinking in Pictures and Other Reports from My Life with Autism,* written by Temple, and *An Anthropologist on Mars: Seven Paradoxical Tales,* by Oliver Sacks, which has a story in it about Temple. Emily recognized a fascinating story. She called Temple's agent. The next thing she knew she was meeting in a restaurant with Temple Grandin, who said yes to making her life story into an HBO movie.

Temple knew Saines's work because she had founded Autism Coalition Resources, which became Autism Speaks. Emily was also a talent agent and felt a responsibility to get the story to the public. "Parents of a child with autism really needed to hear it," said Emily.

Selling a story about an autistic woman who designs slaughterhouses proved to be a long journey. "In one of the first versions of the movie, they wanted me to have a romance," said Temple. "Romance is not in character for me."[2]

Ten years after the project started, the group that made the movie met on the stage at the 2010 Emmy Awards. They had collected awards for best actress, best director, best supporting actor, best supporting actress, and best screenplay. "I absolutely knew a mom would do it right."[3]

"You wouldn't recognize Claire Danes," said Temple.[4] "She became me in the 1960s and 1970s. It was like going into a time machine. I spent a day with her and three days with Mick Jackson, the director. I also was very involved in the accuracy of the cattle." Temple was delighted that they used her plans to recreate the dip vat for the movie.

"Not everybody on the spectrum thinks in pictures, but the movie is clinically accurate for me. It shows my anxiety, which was calmed by the hug machine and a small dose of antidepressant. I don't use the hug machine anymore, but continue to take the antidepressant. Though I deal with them much better now, I still have sensory issues," she continued.[5]

Claire Danes, who played the part of Temple Grandin, had a movement coach and a voice coach. She said, "I worked hard. I was inspired by Temple's courage. I don't expect to have another opportunity for a role this good soon. Temple found a way to self-soothe and now she's capable and formidable. Though she's not cured, she's learned how to cope with her autism. Now, she's quite polished and relates in a more normal way."[6]

Catherine O'Hara, a Canadian-American actress and comedienne, plays Aunt Ann. Ann exposes Temple to cattle for the first time on her Arizona ranch. One scene shows Temple lying on the ground with cows crowding all around her. In another scene with Aunt Ann, Temple, and a horse, Temple reveals her sensitivity to animals. She says, "He's pointing his ears at you, he's looking at you. Now, I've got his attention, he's looking at me."[7]

Mick Jackson, the director, chose Catherine to play Aunt Ann because he wanted to portray a warm, sympathetic person. "If you cast someone who has a comedic career, sometimes they know more about the human condition than a character actor."[8]

David Strathairn portrays Mr. Carlock, Temple's science teacher in middle school and high school. Temple loved science and was an eager pupil. He mentored her and gave her a safe haven from teasing by the other kids. Mr. Carlock was perhaps the first to realize Temple's amazing mind. She literally thought in pictures, able to bring up pictures from all kinds of situations and visualize how things would look.

"The screenwriter and I had decided to call him Dr. Carlock to convey an eminence that would enhance the impression he made on Temple. She thought that giving him his doctorate was a way of giving back thanks for everything he'd done for her," said Jackson.[9]

Julia Ormond, an English actress, played Eustacia, Temple's mother. She won an Emmy. At the Vista Del Mar Autism Conference in Vista Del Mar, California, Julia gifted her Emmy to Eustacia Cutler. "I know that as a young woman Eustacia Cutler's dream was to be an actress," Ormond said. "She put aside her own dream and sacrificed everything for her children. She played the most important role a woman can play in life—that of a loving and caring mother. And for that I want her to have my Emmy."[10]

"You can use it as a doorstop," Ormond said to Eustacia as she presented it to her.[11] Eustacia hugged Ormond and then clutched the Emmy. "The theme of the movie is, 'Follow your gut feeling to help unlock a door for someone like Temple who's locked in,'" said Julia.

The Emmy-award winning screenplay was written by Christopher Monger and William Merritt Johnson. Two groundbreaking books, *Emergence*, written by Temple Grandin and Margaret Scariano, and *Thinking in Pictures*, by Temple Grandin, were used as a basis for the script. Mick Jackson, who has directed many movies, said his favorite among the movies he's directed is *Temple Grandin*.

Jackson said, "Temple had an eye for the details that were right and the details that were wrong, but she also had—unusual for someone whose life you're telling through film—a sense of what it's like to make a movie, to put it together in a whole picture."[12]

Temple called Jackson after the screening, wildly enthusiastic. "I realized that what we'd shown in the movie, which is her being able to run things in her head, was true," Jackson recalled. "She was quoting me shots and edits and things from the movie she'd seen once. She'd downloaded the movie into her head like a DVD, and she was running it forwards and backwards."[13]

Temple had seen an earlier movie directed by Jackson and noticed some problems. "By the time Mick was working on my movie, he knew what his strengths were and where he needed help, so every time Mick wanted to change something in the script, he would consult with one of the writers, Christopher Monger. He was a word thinker, of course, but he was also a pattern thinker who could tell what effect each little change was going to have on the overall structure. The movie benefited enormously from being created by three kinds of thinking."[14]

Temple said the movie is "clinically accurate," so apparently the parts important to her are correct. "People with autism vary from the Silicon Valley genius to the nonverbal. I received fantastic mail from people on all points of the spectrum," Temple said. "There are still lots of people who have never heard of autism. I hope this movie will educate people. The most important message of the movie is that people with autism can do things."[15]

CHAPTER 22

AUTISM IS A FAMILY DISORDER

Autism is a family disorder. This doesn't mean everyone in the family has autism, but if one person has severe autism, the whole family is affected. There's a strong genetic component, so there's a good chance that one or more members of the extended family has Asperger's. The Grandin family pattern—a mother very involved with the autistic child, a distant father who probably had Asperger's, and siblings who don't speak out—is unfortunately very common.

Of all the factors that shape your personality—your genes, your parents, your peers—siblings are at the top, according to one major theory of human development. The relationship with your sisters and brothers will likely last longer than any others in your lifetime. If one of the siblings has autism, it makes a huge impact on the family.

Temple was born on August 29, 1947, in an era when autism was nearly unknown. The second child in the Grandin family was born in May 1949, the third in 1953, and the youngest in June 1955. Four children in eight years. Obviously, they were close in age and undoubtedly did many things together. "Temple is autistic when it suits her to be autistic. And normal when it suits her to be normal," the siblings grumbled. This is a common complaint among siblings.

"A normal child doesn't need to be told that the nonverbal autistic sibling requires more attention from their parents—that, in many ways, the world of the family revolves around that child," wrote Temple.[1] Even a verbal child with autism makes an enormous difference.

Autism affects every aspect of life, but autistics are not all alike. They are all individuals. As the mantra goes, "If you've met one person with autism, you've met one person with autism." Four times as many boys have autism as girls. Autism affects people of all races, incomes, ethnic groups, and religion.

Temple says that fortunately none of her siblings are autistic. She says that her sister, one and a half years younger than she, was the most affected by her autism because Temple got all the attention. Temple was interested in anything that flew—kites, airplanes, rockets. Her sister wanted to be a ballerina, "the last thing I wanted to be," said Temple. The two were in school at the same time so her sister suffered from teasing about "that weird Temple." The younger siblings, who arrived five and six years later, were never in the same school.

Temple's siblings did not attend the awards for the HBO movie, *Temple Grandin,* because they didn't want to be identified.

Dick Grandin, Temple's father, had survived the Battle of the Bulge. He wanted to return to the life he had known in Boston. As a peacetime dad, he had the embarrassing intrusion of a kid who didn't fit in. "Men take autism harder than women. It insults their sense of honor," said Eustacia Cutler at the autism conference I attended. All too common among parents with a child who has autism, Temple's parents divorced when she was a teen. "Fully 80 percent of couples with autistic children break up," says an expert.[2]

Like most autistics, Temple shrank from touch for years. I was startled when I met Natalie, a slim seven-year-old in a sundress, in the waiting room of a busy restaurant. She flitted from person to person hugging everybody. She sometimes said, "I love you." Reactions varied.

I asked her how old she was and where she would be in school. No answer. Her mother volunteered that she would be in first grade in an autism class. Natalie doesn't answer direct questions, but she does interact with others in her own way. It was refreshing to meet a child with autism who hugs everybody.

Natalie's mother divorced Natalie's father and has remarried. Natalie lives with her mother and stepfather. She has no siblings.

I interviewed Tim Carney, Neil Carney's next older brother. Neil was diagnosed with autism at three. Now twenty-two and a student at Wichita State University, Tim was three years old when Neil was born. "I don't remember life before Neil," he said.

Neil and Tim were roommates for twelve years. Neil didn't sleep well. After having Neil for a roommate, Tim can sleep through "almost anything."

"Neil affected our family so much more than we realize," Tim said. "I think it was a greatly positive effect."

Neil's mother told me that she thought the four older kids have much more compassion because of Neil. "They don't want to see anyone made fun of. Neil doesn't understand when he's being made fun of, but they do," she said.

Tim said, "As Neil got older, he got more aggressive. He doesn't like grooming—shaving, trimming nails, getting his hair cut. Neil bit through my shirt and took out a chunk of flesh once when I was trying to help my mother with these necessary tasks.

"Neil can hurt you. You have to be careful," said Tim. "You have to watch Neil 24/7. If you step away, he could disappear. You need to keep eyes on him all the time.

"Our family is extremely blessed. There are four older, responsible kids. Our dad is well-paid. Carneys are well-known in Wichita. Grandpa Carney was the fire chief. Many relatives live in the area. We have literally hundreds of cousins. Our grandparents watched Neil when he was younger. An aunt and uncle watched him, too."

"Neil has no idea how lucky he is," I said. Tim agreed.

Tim told me that the Carney family has unofficially adopted Bethany, Neil's caretaker, as another sibling. She has taken good care of Neil for more than two years. "Bethany is passionate about what she does. We're very thankful to have her," said Martin, the middle Carney child.

"Growing up with Neil was frustrating," said Martin. "He taught me patience, understanding, and not to make judgments. It was a whole family endeavor. I can't help but wonder what's going to happen to Neil when our parents are gone."

"People like Neil open up new ideas. Like maybe I should think about something besides making one hundred thousand dollars a year," said Martin. "Neil has encouraged an interest in psychology. Sometimes I have dreams where Neil was normal.

"I love him, but I realize Neil may not feel love like we do. I have lots of questions. Is Neil happy? What would it be like to have his brain? Does he see colors differently? Hear differently? Are his sensory pathways different?

"When Neil was having chronic rage fits from too much medication, I couldn't imagine being drugged every day and not having the ability to communicate."

Martin admits that Neil is better off now that he's not on so much medication. So is his family. Everyone benefits from Neil's current living situation, in a house with a caregiver.

"How does Neil function? I think it would be cool to do research about this. Neil has helped me with processing, critical skills dissecting. He's been an interesting brother. I wouldn't trade him," Martin said.

"I was lucky to have normal siblings. We shared the experience of Neil together. We talked about Neil."

Rachel Storey is a grandmother whose grandson has Asperger's. She asked, "How much does a grandparent get involved?"

"We discovered Evan had Asperger's between fourth and fifth grades," said Rachel. "My fear was violence. When he got upset, he would double his fists, even at his father. I was afraid he'd hurt somebody. He's always been a big boy. At school one day, they called the police, he was acting out so much. He's always struggled in school, but no one could figure out why he had so much anger.

"When his mother sent him to his room, he took the screens off his bedroom window and escaped, which infuriated her. I knew he needed counseling. The parents said they couldn't afford it. I said I'd pay for it.

"Once he was diagnosed, the blame game began—he didn't get it from my family. My thought was, 'It's here. We're going to deal with it.'

"The counselor at Kansas University taught us how to handle him. He just wanted to go out and walk around. To defuse himself. That's what he does when he gets upset. Now he's allowed to do that.

"When he was in elementary school, he walked the perimeters of the playground. They called him 'The Giant.' All through late elementary school and junior high, a para[professional] sat next to him. He hated it.

"He's always been mainly nonverbal. He frequently answers questions with a shoulder shrug. In a crowd he's not going to say one word. If we're the only ones in the car, Evan and I can have a conversation," said Rachel.

"Evan doesn't like attention. He hates to have happy birthday sung to him. He's tall, six feet and five inches, and he was a good basketball player, but he didn't like being the center of attention, so he quit.

"I'm helping Evan learn to cope with attention," his grandmother said. "He's learning to just say 'thank you' and move on.

"When his sisters are proud of themselves, they talk and talk. One of them got straight A's [during the] last nine weeks, which she'd never done in her life. Finally Evan said, 'You're not the only one that got A's. I got some A's too.'"

Rachel gets tickled when Evan tells them to "cool it." "It's much better than punching them," she said.

Evan's family now understands people with autism. They are much more sensitive and understanding of the condition. And they are extremely proud of Evan, who finished his first year at college and is independent.

Gretchen DiGiovanni, wife of Sean and mother to Sam, Jack, and Paul, is the former director of development at Heartspring in Wichita, Kansas. Sam has autism. Gretchen and Sean knew they wanted children. When no children appeared, Gretchen visited the doctor. "You will have children," he told her, "but it will be in vitro."

The first time Gretchen went to the doctor for a prenatal checkup, he told her she would have twins. "The second time the doctor heard three heartbeats, so we knew early we would be having triplets," said Gretchen.

Jack and Paul are identical. Sam was always a little behind them in development. Sam was a good, cuddly baby—not hypersensitive. His parents thought he was deaf. Sam was formally diagnosed with autism at the age of twenty-five months.

Gretchen belonged to a national triplet mom's group. Of the thirty-five to forty families, 90 percent had some kind of fertility assistance. Quite a high percentage of the triplets have one or more on the spectrum.

"Though we had the advantage of early diagnosis," said Gretchen, "it was a scary time." She was staying home with the boys, working part-time in the business she had worked in formerly.

Now the triplets are thirteen and in the same school. "I would never have dreamed this would be the life we'd live," said Gretchen, "but it's good. Jack and Paul have each other to rely on. They model everything for Sam. Sam's speech is good, but carrying on a conversation is difficult. He imitates TV shows, so he can say anything, but not necessarily know what he's saying. Every month or so, he takes a sudden leap in improvement."

Sam never forgets a teacher, a paraprofessional, or a therapist, and there have been many. The other night he said, "I'm anxious, Mom. I need to go to the North Pole." Recognizing he's anxious is an accomplishment for any thirteen-year-old, let alone one with autism. "That comes from good teachers," said Gretchen. The DiGiovannis recognize there will be many unknown difficulties ahead, but that's parenting.

Autism often impairs one's judgment of what's socially acceptable. Having a sense of humor helps immensely when dealing with this disorder. The Autism Society of the Heartland decided there's enough humor for other people to enjoy, too. They organized a fund-raiser featuring parents giving comic routines about some of the incidents they'd experienced.

Chris Long told a story about going to McDonald's with her husband Scott and their eleven-year-old autistic son Dakota. Although Dakota doesn't talk, he loves to rub people's skin.

"He'll rub your arms or your back," she said. "Any warm skin. He just loves it. So we're at McDonald's Play Place and he's doing great. But pretty soon he starts rubbing this lady's arm and she's turning redder and redder.

"It's summertime and she's got this huge chest, and a very low-cut top. Dakota reaches in and grabs the woman's boob and starts rubbing. I don't know what to do. I'm like, 'Scott?' And he's like, 'What? You want me to grab the other one?'"

A grandmother told me that her mildly autistic grandson loved touching black fabric. Since many people wear black clothing, this could present some embarrassing situations. Many servers in restaurants wear black, as well as numerous people just walking down the street. Just imagine the problems with an obsession about touching black material could cause!

Family members find themselves in unusual situations: funny, stressful, and sometimes awe-inspiring. Here are some helpful suggestions for dealing with these situations.

Acknowledge feelings: Parents will feel shock, depression, guilt, anger, sadness, and anxiety. So will the siblings. With fewer life experiences, young people will be less prepared to cope with their emotions. Simple acknowledgement on an age-appropriate level can help. If life seems too difficult, some families will want to consult a professional.

Hold family discussions: Discuss problems openly in the family. Encourage questions and reactions. A disability needs to be talked about. In my family, lack of communication made understanding and living with my sister more difficult. Avoiding dialogue will only encourage hiding problems when family members are adults with families of their own. Children know the secrets of their parents. They know that something important is not being shared and cannot interpret the feeling that something is terribly wrong.

Keep informed: As parents learn about autism, so should other family members on an age-appropriate level.

Encourage everyone to go on after an embarrassing situation: Tiffany experienced many of these while growing up with her sister, Lindsay, who has severe autism. Once, when the girls were very young, they were in church singing, "Lord, have mercy." Lindsay suddenly burst out screaming, "Oh, no, we're all going to hell." Her mother hastily took her out of church. Tiffany said, "For the good of everyone, forgive, learn from the situation, and go on."

Have a sense of humor: This does not mean to make fun of the person with a disability or laugh at her. However, laughter helps. Ciara chose her disabled brother to attend the guest book at her wedding. "I chose him because I love him," Ciara said. She worked with him for months on what to say: "Welcome to Ciara's wedding. Sign the book." What he actually said was, "You're late. Go home." "You have to have a sense of humor," said Ciara. "He's kept his through all that's happened to him."

Find a friend whose sibling also has special needs: Gordon, who's seventeen, has a twelve-year-old brother with autism. He made a friend, the drummer of a band he plays in, whose brother is also in special education. "No one else knows what it's like to have a brother with disabilities except my best friend," Gordon said.

Promote an attitude of gratitude: Everyone has his own idea of thankfulness. At the age of three, my brother said, "Thank you, God, for green beanz, pork'n beanz, and all other else beanz." Though I like beans, this would probably not be my top priority in the thankfulness department. I don't do it daily, but I keep a gratitude journal. In the journal I write down five things I'm thankful for and date it. When I look back, I am reminded of what was happening on that day, as well as many blessings. There's nothing magic about the number five. Two or ten will do as well.

Join a group: They provide support and information. Some suggestions: Autism Speaks, National Autism Society, and Autism Society of America.

Read: I've done a lot of this. There are lots of books about autism. Some of my favorites are *The Horse Boy* by Rupert Isaacson, *Elijah's Cup* by Valerie Paradiž, and Temple Grandin's *Autistic Brain*.

Use the Internet: Use the information. Visit blogs. New sites pop up all the time. Admittedly, some information on the web is worthless. Sharing with someone who has the same concerns is priceless.

Stay open to possibilities: Things are happening to benefit persons with autism and their family members all the time. What is known today is different from what was known ten years ago or even one year ago. Who knows what will be discovered tomorrow?

CHAPTER 23

AUTISM IS IN YOUR BRAIN

In the last ten years we've learned more about the inner workings of the brain than we've learned throughout the history of civilization.

"In the ancient world, physicians believed that the brain was made of phlegm," writes Carl Zimmer in his article "Secrets of the Brain." "Aristotle looked on it as a refrigerator, cooling off the fiery heart. From his time through the Renaissance, anatomists declared with great authority that our perceptions, emotions, reasoning, and actions were all the result of 'animal spirits'—mysterious, unknowable vapors that swirled through cavities in our head and traveled through our bodies.

"The scientific revolution in the seventeenth century began to change that. The British physician Thomas Willis recognized that the custard-like tissue of the brain was where our mental world existed. To understand how it worked, he dissected brains of sheep, dogs and expired patients, producing the first accurate maps of the organ."[1]

In the twenty-first century our interest has accelerated, especially since we have equipment that shows more details.

In April 2013, President Obama declared a federal brain mapping project aimed at conquering challenges such as autism, Alzheimer's, and epilepsy. He called it Brain Research Through Advancing Neurotechnologies (BRAIN). Experts hope such efforts will advance the fight against autism, Alzheimer's, and epilepsy. It will take decades.

"Neuroscience is arguably the hottest field in science these days, and we'd be foolish not to try to take advantage of the potential it offers," said science budget expert Al Teich of George Washington University's Center for International Science and Technology Policy.[2]

Much interest has turned to understanding the neurological condition of autism. This is a priority since autism numbers continue to rise. "We still don't have a litmus test for autism," said the neuroscientist Joy Hirsch, director of the Functional MRI Research Center at the Columbia Medical Center. "But we have a basis for it."[3] One review article summarized: "This body of research clearly established autism and its signs and symptoms as being of neurologic origin."[4]

Autism really is in your brain.

Because Temple Grandin is such a well-known person with autism, many scientists have wanted to scan her brain for research. Seven or eight times Temple has stayed quite still in a large cylinder, waiting with anticipation for the racket to be over, while her brain was scanned.

Temple was one of the first autistic subjects to undergo magnetic resonance imaging, or MRI. Her first brain scan was in 1987 at the University of California, Santa Barbara.

She immediately noticed that a ventricle on the left side was much longer than the one on the right.

At the University of Utah in 2010, neuroscientist Jason Cooperrider and colleagues scanned Grandin's brain using three different methods: high-resolution MRI, which captures the structure of the brain; diffusion tensor imaging (DTI), a method to trace the connections between brain regions; and functional MRI, which indicates brain activity.

Functional MRI is a type of specialized brain and body scan used to map neural activity in the brain by imaging the change in blood flow related to energy use by brain cells. Since the early 1990s, functional MRI has come to dominate brain mapping research.

Temple's left ventricle is 57 percent larger than her right, as showed by a University of Utah study. In control subjects the difference between left and right was only 15 percent.

"Back in 1987, neuroimaging technology wasn't capable of measuring the anatomical structures within the brain with great precision. But if the researchers had known that one ventricle was 7,093 millimeters long while the other was 3,868 millimeters long, it would have given them pause."[5]

The University of Utah scans also showed that Grandin's amygdala, which plays an important role in emotional processing, is larger than normal. This helps explain why she feels so much fear and anxiety.

"I want to emphasize that not everyone with autism has such a large amygdala," said Temple. "Mine is three times as large as normal. The brain scan shows what showed up in the classroom and in life.

"I *like* knowing that my high level of anxiety might be related to having an enlarged amygdala. The problem isn't *out there*, the problem is *in here*, the way I'm wired. The threat isn't real. The feeling of the threat is."[6]

"Researchers can't be sure that an anomaly in one brain will have the same effect in a different brain. Just because you have an enlarged amygdala doesn't mean you're autistic,"

Temple wrote.[7] And not all autistic brains are alike. What's in one autistic brain is not the same as what's in someone else's autistic brain.

Thomas Insel, director of the National Institute of Mental Health, told *USA Today* in 2012, "Even when you look at a child who has no language, who is self-injuring, who has had multiple seizures, you would be amazed at how normal their brains look. It's the most inconvenient truth about this condition."[8]

HDFT (high-definition fiber tracking) was underwritten by the Department of Defense to investigate traumatic brain injuries. "They came to me saying we need something for brain injury like what X-rays do for orthopedic injury," said Dr. Walter Schneider, professor of psychology and senior scientist at the Learning Development and Research Center (LRDC) and professor of neurosurgery at the University of Pennsylvania.

"Just like there are 2,006 bones in your body, there are major cables in your brain," Dr. Schneider says. "You can ask most anybody on the street to create a drawing of what a broken bone looks like, and they would be able to draw something somewhat sensible. If you ask them, 'So what does a broken brain look like?' most people, including researchers in the field, couldn't do it."[9]

Temple has learned a lot from various scans. "Autistic brains aren't broken," said Temple. "My own brain isn't broken. My circuits aren't broken. They just didn't grow properly.

"I know that my cerebellum is 20 percent smaller than the norm. The cerebellum helps control motor coordination, so this abnormality probably explains why my sense of balance is lousy."[10]

It's remarkable what it can tell you, but HDFT can't tell what you're thinking or feeling or what political opinions you have. HDFT can't solve all the mysteries of the brain.

Temple often compares her brain with a search engine. When Dr. Schneider showed her images from her HDFT scan at the University of Pittsburg in 2012, Temple said, "Oh, you found my search engine."[11]

She said that the original search engines were probably designed by people whose brains work like hers—"people with brains that have trouble with linear thought, brains that ramble, brains that have weak short-term memory."[12]

The brain is amazing, and we still have lots to learn about it. Eleanor Maguire, a British neuroscientist, did a study in England in 2000 on taxi drivers that showed using your brain helps it grow.

She looked at the MRIs of the hippocampi of sixteen licensed London cabbies. The hippocampus is believed to house three types of cells that help us navigate: place cells, which recognize landmarks; head direction cells, which tell you which way you're facing; and grid cells, which tell you where you are in relation to where you've been. What Maguire found was that the hippocampi of drivers who had mastered the "knowledge"—the location of every nook in the city and the quickest way to get there—were larger than those of control subjects.[13]

The longer the driver stayed on the job, the larger his hippocampus. When he left the job, his hippocampus returned to normal.

"The brain behaves like a muscle," Maguire said. "Use brain regions and they grow."[14]

If you don't use a brain region, it doesn't necessarily wither. Even though they can't see, blind persons use the visual cortex to navigate. Temple had a blind roommate when she was in high school.

Temple said, "'I called her a 'cane master.' She didn't want a guide dog leading her. She wanted to learn how to guide herself. And boy, did she ever. She needed to be walked through a new environment only once, and then she knew her way. Outside our dorm was a busy intersection; she navigated it as well as any sighted person. Maybe she wasn't using actual images, but her *visual* cortex was allowing her to build a vivid, knowable, and navigable world."[15]

Mark Deesing, Temple Grandin's assistant, explains how Temple's method of keeping information straight reflects how her brain works.

"Temple keeps her calendar on an old-fashioned paper, one with big boxes. She has ten pages of phone call notes a day, scribbled in little handwriting only she can read. She fills in her whole schedule, names, contact information, flight numbers, and so on into that box.

"She takes apart the calendar and zeroes it, then staples it together. She keeps her calendar every year and knows just where to get it. One drawer has several million bits of information and she can find it just like that.

"Her filing system is similar to how her brain works. Pictures with text that trigger information. Each box is compact. She recalls the data completely."[16]

Brain wiring also affects the ability to handle transitions. People with autism can have trouble with even simple transitions. The brain seems to become overwhelmed.

"Temple talked, for example, about how difficult it is to transition from one sensory mode to another, like switching from visual to auditory awareness," says Valerie Paradiž in *Elijah's Cup*. "The world for an autistic person is a highly fragmented place, and any traditional cohesion it might have is constructed through a long and arduous process of piecing together disparate sensory elements.

"Not only does Temple's thinking go from specific to general, so do her emotions and social behaviors. She was able, over the course of many years, to integrate various functions that most of us take for granted. She did it by accessing a vast catalogue of images she had built up in her mind: 'This thing that people call thought, facts and emotions all merged together . . . I don't have that. My memory works like slides. I speed-search the Internet. If I hold it up on the screen in my mind, it turns into a video. Then it gets sound, and then it gets emotion. But they don't all come up together.'"[17]

Sensory sensitivities are a well-known aspect of an autistic brain.

"Autistic brains, it turns out, have a much greater number of nerve cells than 'neurotypical' brains," says Rupert Isaacson, author of *Horse Boy*. "The result can be extreme sensory overload. . . .The fluorescent lights of a supermarket or daycare facility could look like lights being strobed at one million times a second."[18]

Researchers are constantly working on studies that will be helpful to persons with autism. Occasionally, there's a breakthrough.

In August 2014, Michael Halassa, principal investigator and New York University Langone Medical Center assistant professor, published a study in *Cell*. It noted that "The brain juggles two different sets of information. Input from the world around you, like sights and sounds, has to be processed. But so does internal information—your memories and thoughts."[19]

Some people, especially persons with autism and schizophrenia, have difficulty knowing what is occurring internally and what is occurring externally. Researchers observed the switching mechanism in mice for the first time. Halassa said, "This is going to translate to humans." He and other researchers will try to find the same mechanism in people. If they find it, the result could be a range of treatments for persons with varying degrees of severity in autism and schizophrenia.

Brains are wired differently. Some people respond much more readily to social information while others—like scientists, researchers, and engineers—key in on details. "We need detail-oriented people in this world or there would be no electricity, cars, or beautiful works of music," said Temple. "Detail-oriented engineers make sure the lights stay on and the bridges do not fall down."[20]

Temple is confident there are design miscalculations she wouldn't make. "I use object visual thinking so I'm able to *see* a catastrophe before it happens," she says.[21] She says she could have foreseen the Fukushima nuclear power plant accident in 2011. "Where was the backup located? In the basement of a nuclear power plant that is located next to the sea. As I read many descriptions of the accident, I could see the water flowing into the plant, and I could see the emergency generators disappearing under the water."[22]

Temple says, "Everyone in life has a different set of strengths and challenges within a unique personality. I am a pure techie and having a good career gives my life meaning. I've learned to make the most of the way my brain is hardwired and I don't feel remorse over missing cables in the social parts of my brain."[23]

CHAPTER 24

TEMPLE GRANDIN'S LEGACY

Temple Grandin's favorite quote is by Alan Ashley Pitt: "The man who follows the crowd will usually get no further than the crowd. The man who walks alone is likely to find himself in places no one has ever been before."

Temple has been a mold-breaker and an important role model for educators, parents, and those with mild autism. She's also explained autism from the inside, but her autism remains secondary. "Don't focus so much on autism that you forget everything else," Temple says. She certainly follows her own advice.

Though born with severe autism, Temple has become a beacon of hope for those with autism. "Temple broke through the barriers of autism to show that people with autism and Asperger's add value to our society," said Dr. Kurt Vogel of the University of Wisconsin in River Falls, one of Temple's former students.

Temple has written several books for persons with autism and those interested in the subject. She wrote *Emergence: Labeled Autistic; Thinking in Pictures and Other Reports from My Life with Autism; The Way I See It: A Personal Look at Autism and*

Asperger's; The Unwritten Rules of Social Relationships: Decoding Social Mysteries Through the Unique Perspectives of Autism with Sean Barron; and *The Autistic Brain: Helping Different Kinds of Minds Succeed* with Richard Panek.

A highly acclaimed speaker about autism, Temple's TED Talk, "The World Needs All Kinds of Minds," in February 2010 has subtitles available in thirty-six languages.

Temple is known worldwide for overcoming the challenges of autism, but her primary identity isn't autism. She thinks of herself as an expert on livestock, a scientist, and a professor.

"Temple has been to domestic animals what Jane Goodall has been to primates," said Dr. Bernard Rollin of Colorado State University.

Temple stresses measurement in her work with livestock. She measures the number of moos (cattle that moo and bellow, no more than 3 percent) and the number of falls (cattle that fall, no more than 1 percent). She trains others to stick to definite standards, too. Because of her autism, Temple doesn't understand abstract ideas, but she's used this to her advantage and that of animals. She stresses what you can and should test. Ironically, many of the things important to her career—hard work, persistence, and insight—are not measurable.

Conditions for animals have much improved because of Temple's requirements. "Audits required by McDonald's, Whole Foods, and other companies have forced plant management to monitor, measure, and improve employee behavior. Plants are maintaining their equipment better and reassigning/firing employees who abuse animals," reports Temple.[1]

Especially for women, she created jobs. "Until I came along, secretaries were the only women in this industry," said Temple. "I opened many jobs for females in the cattle industry."

Temple has provided many tools for progressive practices using principles from scientific literature and personal experience. "If the animals on America's factory farms got together to award an Animal Nobel Prize, they would surely give it to Temple Grandin," says Michael Pollan, author of *In Defense of Food.*

In August 2014, Temple attended the sixtieth International Congress of Meat Science and Technology in Punta Del Este, Uruguay. She was one of five hundred participants from more than fifty countries. Temple spoke at the conference, one of thirty-one national and international speakers recognized worldwide to speak. She continues to speak at conferences around the world, spreading her expertise on livestock.

Temple also defines herself as a scientist. "For a scientist, the lack of knowledge is thrilling. A new field to explore. A chance to do fundamental, big-picture research before the field gets really narrow and specialized! Questions that lead to other questions! What could be more fun?" she asked.[2]

Science has fascinated Temple since childhood. In grade school, she flew kites behind her bicycle that she had cut from a single sheet of heavy drawing paper. She discovered that bending the tips of the wings up made the kite fly higher. The same design started making appearances in commercial aircraft thirty years later.

In high school, she used science to develop the squeeze machine after researching principles of sensory interaction. Her science teacher, Mr. Carlock, encouraged her to do research. She's been intrigued with science since then. She considers herself a totally logical and scientific person.

One of Temple's idols is Albert Einstein. He said, "Science without religion is lame. Religion without science is blind." Temple said, "Both are needed to answer life's great questions."

"I continually add to my library of knowledge and constantly update both my scientific knowledge and my beliefs about God. It is beyond my comprehension to accept anything on faith alone," said Temple.[3]

In *The Autistic Brain*, Temple showed her willingness not only to study science, but also to allow scientists to study her brain. As she has done many times, Temple shared the results with us, opening herself to the world.

"Perhaps in the future," said Dr. Simon Baron-Cohen, a leading autism expert in Cambridge, England, "it is going to be increasingly controversial whether autism is something that needs to be cured or not. Perhaps it is more a personality type."[4] Temple would certainly agree with that.

Temple also defines herself as a professor, and her colleagues and students agree that she is both effective and beloved.

"Temple has affected me very deeply. Temple and I share a passion for teaching," said Dr. Kurt Vogel of the University of Wisconsin. "It's unusual for someone of her stature to concentrate so much on teaching.

"Because she understands them, Temple uses word pictures in her teaching. During the 2008 financial bailout, she said that the bailout cost approximately two Denver airports for every state in the union. The Denver airport cost almost $5 billion." Her unique way of thinking and teaching resonates with her students.

"She's much beloved by her students. She's utterly devoted to them. They follow her around like puppy dogs," said Bernard Rollin.

"Temple puts her students above her work," said Mark Deesing. "She has dozens of students imprinted with Temple Grandin ideas out there." She's given seminars in many other countries, so she has spread her ideas to students across the world.

"I want to inspire students to make a positive difference," said Temple. "I hope they will do well."

Undoubtedly, through her expertise on animals, scientific accomplishments, and success as a professor, Temple will get the permanent recognition she longs for.

ENDNOTES

Chapter 1

1. Eustacia Cutler, *A Thorn in My Pocket: Temple Grandin's Mother Tells the Family Story*, Arlington, Texas: Future Horizons, 2004, 195.
2. Ibid, 11.
3. Ibid, 9.
4. Ibid, 9.
5. Battle of the Bulge, Wikipedia.com.
6. *A Thorn in My Pocket*, 12.
7. Ibid, 25.
8. Dr. Temple Grandin and Sean Barron, *The Unwritten Rules of Social Relationships: Decoding Social Mysteries Through the Unique Perspectives of Autism*, Arlington, Texas: Future Horizons, 2005, 38.
9. Ibid, 39.
10. Temple Grandin, PhD, *The Way I See It: A Personal Look at Autism and Asperger's*, Arlington, Texas: Future Horizons, 2008, 26.
11. Ibid, 232.
12. Ibid, 46.
13. *Social Relationships*, 11.
14. Temple Grandin, *Thinking in Pictures and Other Reports from My Life with Autism*, New York: Doubleday, 1995, 20.
15. Temple Grandin, PhD, and Margaret Scariano, *Emergence: Labeled Autistic*, London: , 1986, 43.
16. Ibid, 58.
17. *Emergence*, 39.

18. Ibid, 39.
19. Naoki Higashida, *The Reason I Jump*, New York: Random House, 2013, 24.
20. Temple Grandin and Richard Panek, *The Autistic Brain: Helping Different Kinds of Minds Succeed*, New York: Houghton Mifflin Harcourt, 2013, 9.

Chapter 2

1. Temple Grandin and Catherine Johnson, *Animals in Translation: Using the Mysteries of Autism to Decode Animal Behavior*, New York: Harcourt, 2006, 3.
2. *Emergence*, 75.
3. *Thinking in Pictures*, 78.
4. *The Way I See It*, 48.
5. *Thinking in Pictures*, 101.
6. *Autistic Brain*, 183.
7. *A Thorn in My Pocket*, 184.
8. *Emergence*, 84.
9. Ibid, 85.
10. *Thinking in Pictures*, 175.
11. Sy Montgomery, *Temple Grandin: How the Girl Who Loved Cows Embraced Autism and Changed the World*, New York: Houghton Mifflin Harcourt, 2012, 61.
12. *The Way I See It*, 231.
13. *Emergence*, 95.
14. Ibid, 113.

Chapter 3

1. *Thinking in Pictures*, 104.
2. *Autistic Brain*, 108.
3. Richard Pollak, *The Creation of Doctor B: A Biography of Bruno Bettelheim*, New York: Simon & Schuster, 1998, 272.
4. Ibid, 278.
5. Ibid, 279.
6. Ibid, 282.
7. Ibid, 282.
8. *Emergence*, 113.

9.   Ibid, 117.

Chapter 4

1.   *Thinking in Pictures*, 104.
2.   *Emergence*, 128.
3.   *Animals in Translation*, 51.
4.   Valerie Paradiž, *Elijah's Cup: A Family's Journey into the Community and Culture of High-Functioning Autism and Asperger's Syndrome*, New York: Free Press, 2002, 69.
5.   Dr. Temple Grandin, "Making the Transition from the World of School to the World of Work," Autism Research Institute.
6.   *Autistic Brain*, 171.
7.   *Social Relationships*, 31.
8.   *The Way I See It*, 217.
9.   *Thinking in Pictures*, 22.
10. Sy Montomery, *Temple Grandin*, 92.
11. Ibid, 94.
12. Temple Grandin, "Successful Technology Transfer of Behavioral and Animal Welfare Research to the Farm and Slaughter Plant," *Improving Animal Welfare: A Practical Approach*, Oxfordshire, UK: CABI, 2010, 216.
13. *The Way I See It*, 20.
14. *Social Relationships*, 25.
15. "Making the Transition from the World of School to the World of Work," Autism Research Institute.
16. *The Way I See It*, 236.

Chapter 5

1.   Temple Grandin and Kate Duffy, *Developing Talents: Careers for Individuals with Asperger Syndrome and High-Functioning Autism*, Lenexa, KS: AAPC, 2004, 149.
2.   *Emergence*, 146.
3.   *Improving Animal Welfare*, 68.
4.   *Emergence*, 148.
5.   *The Way I See It*, 171.
6.   Ibid, 162.
7.   Ibid, 145.

8. Ibid, 94.
9. *The Way I See It*, foreword, xiv.
10. Ibid, xv.
11. Oliver Sacks, *An Anthropologist on Mars: Seven Paradoxical Tales*, New York: Knopf, 1995, 274.
12. *Emergence*, 147.
13. *Emergence*, foreword, 2.
14. *Emergence*, preface, 7.
15. Temple Grandin and Catherine Johnson, *Animals Make Us Human: Creating the Best Life for Animals*, New York: Mariner Books, 2010, acknowledgements, 305.
16. *Animals Make Us Human*, 11.
17. Ibid, 173.

Chapter 6

1. Temple Grandin, PhD, "Calming Effects of Deep Touch Pressure in Patients with Autistic Disorder, College Students, and Animals," *Journal of Child* and *Adolescent Psychopharmacology*, Volume 2, Number 1, 1992, Mary Ann Liebert Publishers.
2. *Emergence*, 121.
3. "Calming Effects of Deep Pressure."
4. *Social Relationships*, 32.
5. Temple Grandin, *Livestock Handling and Transport*, Oxfordshire, UK: CABI, 1993, 116.
6. Temple Grandin and Mark J. Deesing, *Genetics and the Behavior of Domestic Animals*, Cambridge, Mass: Academic Press, 1997, 319.
7. Ibid, 330.
8. *An Anthropologist on Mars*, 286.
9. *Thinking in Pictures*, 89.
10. Ibid, 103.
11. *An Anthropologist on Mars*, 261.
12. *Thinking in Pictures*, 132.
13. Ibid, 180.
14. Ibid, 141.
15. *Social Relationships*, 41.

Chapter 7

1. Tribute to Temple Grandin, Colorado State University, October 6, 2004.
2. Temple Grandin, "Thinking in Pictures," Penny W. Stamps Series, University of Michigan, Sept. 9, 2010.
3. *Autistic Brain*, 88.
4. Ibid, 89.
5. Ibid, 89.
6. Ibid, 89.

Chapter 8

1. Temple Grandin, *New York Magazine*.
2. Temple Grandin and Richard Panek, "What's Right with the Autistic Mind," *Time*, October 7, 2013.
3. *Autistic Brain*, 131.
4. Ibid, 76.
5. Ibid, 72.
6. Ibid, 72.
7. *The Way I See It*, 6.
8. Ibid, 70.
9. *Autistic Brain*, 35.
10. *The Way I See It*, 57.
11. *Animals in Translation*, 51.
12. Ibid, 67.
13. *Autistic Brain*, 188.
14. Ibid, 181.

Chapter 9

1. V. S. Ramachandran and Sandra Blakeslee, *Phantoms in the Brain: Probing the Mysteries of the Human Mind*, New York: William Morrow, 1999, 152.
2. *Anthropologist on Mars*, 287.
3. Verlyn Klinkenborg, "What Do Animals Think?" *Discover*, May 2005.
4. *A Thorn in My Pocket*, 167.
5. Ibid, 209.

6. Ibid, 115.
7. *The Way I See It*, 19.
8. Ibid, 115.
9. Ibid, 4.

Chapter 10

1. Norm Ledgin, *Diagnosing Jefferson: Evidence of a Condition That Guided His Beliefs, Behavior, and Personal Associations*, Arlington, TX: Future Horizons, 2000, iv.
2. Ibid, 243.
3. Personal communication with Norm Ledgin.
4. Norm Ledgin, *Asperger's and Self-Esteem: Insight and Hope through Famous Role Models*, Arlington, TX: Future Horizons, 2002, 35.

Chapter 11

1. *Heartspring's Dialogue*, November 2010.

Chapter 12

1. James Poniewozik, "Mourn the Loss," *Time* Commemorative Issue, 2011.
2. Walter Isaacson, *Steve Jobs*, New York: Simon and Schuster, 2011, 82.
3. Ibid, 82.
4. Ibid, 548.
5. Lev Grossman, "Reinventing the Inventor," *Time*, Nov. 18, 2011.
6. *Autistic Brain*, 77.
7. *A Full Life with Autism*, 2012, 39.
8. Ibid, 39.
9. *The Reason I Jump*, 8.
10. Ibid, 9.

Chapter 13

1. *Animals in Translation*, 192.
2. Ibid, 192.
3. *Emergence*, 178.

4. *Autistic Brain*, prologue, viii.

Chapter 14

1. *Animals in Translation*, 12.
2. Ibid, 307.
3. *Thinking in Pictures*, 155.
4. Michael Pollan, "Power Steer," *New York Times*, March 31, 2002.

Chapter 15

1. Temple Grandin with Mark Deesing, *Humane Livestock Handling: Understanding Livestock Behavior and Building Facilities for Healthier Animals*, North Adams, MA: Storey Publishing, 2008, 1.
2. Ibid, 2.
3. *Improving Animal Welfare*, 71.
4. *Humane Livestock Handling*, 1.
5. Verlyn Klinkenborg, "What Do Animals Think?" *Discover*, May 2005.
6. *Improving Animal Welfare*, 67.
7. Ibid, 71.
8. Ibid, 58.
9. *Thinking in Pictures*, 150.
10. *Improving Animal Welfare*, 219.
11. Ibid, 217.
12. "What Do Animals Think?"
13. *Animals Make Us Human*, 174.
14. Ibid, 189.
15. *Genetics and the Behavior of Domestic Animals*, edited by Temple Grandin and Mark Deesing, Second Edition, Cambridge, MA: Academic Press, 2014, 402.
16. *Animals Make Us Human*, 176
17. Dan Voorhis, Big AG is Altering Care for Livestock Spurred by Activists, the *Wichita Eagle*, June 10, 2014.
18. *Livestock Handling and Transportation*, 218.
19. Ibid, 224.

For more information: Glass Walls Project of the American Meat Industry Video Tour of Beef Farm and Processing Plant featuring Temple Grandin, August 23, 2012. Also a Glass Walls Project of the

Meat Industry Video Tour of Pork Farm and Processing Plant featuring Temple Grandin on May 23, 2013. Check online.

Chapter 16

1. *Temple Grandin*, 12.
2. Ibid, 107.
3. *Animals Make Us Human*, 211.
4. *Improving Animal Welfare*, 27.
5. *Genetics and the Behavior of Domestic Animals*, 435.
6. *Animals Make Us Human*, 217.
7. *Improving Animal Welfare*, 27.
8. *Genetics, and the Behavior of Domestic Animals*, 435.
9. Ibid, 435.
10. Ibid, 436.
11. *Improving Animal Welfare*, 27.
12. *Animals Make Us Human*, 222.
13. Ibid, 222.
14. Ibid, 222.
15. *Improving Animal Welfare*, 218.
16. Ibid, 215.
17. *Animals Make Us Human*, 228.
18. *Improving Animal Welfare*, 214.
19. Ibid, 218.
20. Ibid, 3.
21. Mark Deesing, personal communication.
22. *Animals Make Us Human*, 229.
23. Jonathan Frey, "A Five Step Plan to Feed the World," *National Geographic*, May 2014.
24. *Livestock Handling and Transportation*, 355.

Chapter 17

1. *Improving Animal Welfare*, 294.
2. *Animals in Translation*, 67.
3. Ibid, 281.
4. Sy Montgomery, *Temple Grandin, How the Girl Who Loved Cows Embraced Change and Changed the World*, Boston: HMH Books, 2012,
5. *Animals in Translation*, 53.

6.   Ibid, 53.
7.   Ibid, 53.
8.   Ibid, 110.

Chapter 18

1.   Helen Piers, *Taking Care of Your Rabbit (A Young Pet Owner's Guide)*, New York: Barron's Educational Series, 1992, 4.
2.   Ibid, 5.
3.   Mark Evans, *A Practical Guide to Caring for Your Rabbit*, New York: DK Publishing, 1992, 16.
4.   Judith Heneghan, *Love Your Rabbit (Your Perfect Pet)*, New York: Windmill Books, 2013, 10.
5.   Kelley MacAulay and Bobbie Kalman, *Rabbits*, New York: Pet Care (Crabtree Publishing Company), 2005, 24.
6.   *Taking Care of Your Rabbit*, 21.

Chapter 19

1.   "Bengal Cat Cares for Autistic Boy," YouTube, March 10, 2010.
2.   *Animals Make Us Human*, 76.
3.   Ibid, 25.
4.   *Animals in Translation*, 290.
5.   *Elijah's Cup*, 194.
6.   Ibid, 194.
7.   "Service Dogs and Autism," *Asperger's Digest*, March/April 2011.
8.   Ibid.

Chapter 20

1.   *Animals Make Us Human*, 120.
2.   Rupert Isaacson, *The Horse Boy: A Father's Quest to Heal His Son*, New York: Little, Brown & Co, 2009, 59.
3.   "Horseback Riding as Autism Therapy," *Autism Speaks*, March 8, 2013.
4.   Ibid.
5.   *Animals Make Us Human*,120.
6.   *Animals in Transition*, 5.
7.   *Animals Make Us Human*, 119.

8. Ibid, 119.
9. *Animals Make Us Human*, 106.
10. Ibid, 115.
11. Ibid, 111.
12. Ibid, 120.
13. Kathy Nunemaker with Lois Hickman, "Therapeutic Horseback Riding: A Speech Therapist's Experience," Niwot Associated Therapists.
14. Ibid.
15. Ibid.

Chapter 21

1. "Autistic Woman's Story Is Emmy Gold," ABCNews.com, Nov. 3, 2010.
2. "Real Temple Grandin at 2010 Emmy Awards," TV Legends.org, Nov. 17, 2010.
3. Ibid.
4. Ibid.
5. Ibid.
6. Ibid.
7. "His Ears," muchasMovie, 12/13/2010.
8. Will Harris, "Chat with Mick Jackson, director of *Temple Grandin* movie," PremiumHollywood.com, Feb. 5, 2010.
9. Ibid.
10. "Julia Ormond Gives Emmy to Mother of Temple Grandin," Vistadelmar.org, Nov. 18, 2010.
11. Vistadelmar.org, Nov. 19, 2010.
12. "Chat with Mick Jackson," director of Temple Grandin movie, posted by Will Harris, Feb. 5, 2011.
13. Ibid.
14. *Autistic Brain*, 197.
15. "Real Temple Grandin at 2010 Emmy Awards."

Chapter 22

1. *Autistic Brain*, 71.
2. *The Horse Boy*, 47.

Chapter 23

1. Carl Zimmer, "Secrets of the Brain," *National Geographic*, Feb. 2014.
2. Dan Vergana, "Obama Calls for Brain Mapping Project," *USA Today*, April 2, 2013.
3. *Autistic Brain*, 38.
4. Ibid, 34.
5. Ibid, 29
6. Ibid, 38.
7. Ibid, 34.
8. Ibid, 35.
9. Ibid, 42.
10. Ibid, 27.
11. Ibid, 127.
12. Ibid, 126.
13. Ibid, 175.
14. Ibid, 175.
15. Ibid, 178.
16. Personal communication.
17. *Elijah's Cup*, 194.
18. *The Horse Boy*, 19.
19. Rachel Feltman, "A Switchboard in the Brain Could Unlock Treatments for Autism and Schizophrenia," *The Washington Post*, Aug. 14, 2014.
20. *The Way I See It*, 185.
21. *Autistic Brain*, 168.
22. Ibid, 169.
23. *The Way I See It*, 185.

Chapter 24

1. *Animals Make Us Human*, 172.
2. *Autistic Brain*, 63.
3. *Thinking in Pictures*, 89.
4. *The Horse Boy*, 345.

ACKNOWLEDGMENTS

Thanks to the many people who helped with this book. Phyllis Rowland and her writing critique group helped immensely in the early stages. My later editors were Delores Smith and Denise Douty. Thanks too, to the people I interviewed: Mark Deesing, Martin Carney, Tim Carney, Aldona Carney, Terry Dear, Cheryl Miller, Connie Erbert, Kathy Nunemaker, Dr. Conny Flörcke, Dr. Kurt Vogel, Jim Uhl, Dr. Bernard Rollin, Dr. Wendy Fulwider, and of course Dr. Temple Grandin. Last but not least my mentor, Mary McHugh.